MA

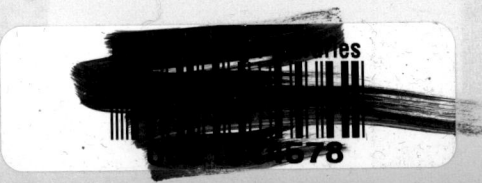

Other books in this series:

Angina
Arthritis
Asthma
Bowel Cancer
Breast Cancer
Chronic Fatigue
Dementia
Depression
Diabetes
High Blood Pressure
How to Stay Healthy
How to Stop Smoking
Irritable Bowel Syndrome
Menopause
Osteoporosis

AB		MO	
MA		MR	
MB		MT	
MC		MW	
MD			
ME			
MG			
MH			
MM			
MN			

Strokes

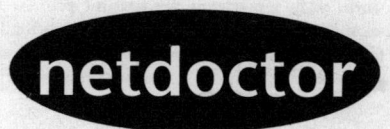

Series Editor
Dr Dan Rutherford
www.netdoctor.co.uk

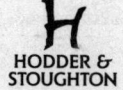

The material in this book is in no way intended to replace professional medical care or attention by a qualified practitioner. The materials in this book cannot and should not be used as a basis for diagnosis or choice of treatment.

Copyright © 2006 by NetDoctor.co.uk
Illustrations copyright © by Amanda Williams

First published in Great Britain in 2006

The right of NetDoctor.co.uk to be identified as the Author of the Work has been asserted by them in accordance with the Copyright, Designs and Patents Act 1988.

All rights reserved. No part of this publication may be reproduced, stored in a retrieval system or transmitted, in any form or by any means, without the prior written permission of the publisher, nor be otherwise circulated in any form of binding or cover other than that in which it is published and without a similar condition being imposed on the subsequent purchaser.

British Library Cataloguing in Publication Data
A record for this book is available from the British Library

ISBN 0 340 862734

Typeset in Garamond by Avon DataSet Ltd,
Bidford-on-Avon, Warwickshire

Printed and bound in Great Britain by
Bookmarque Ltd, Croydon, Surrey

The paper and board used in this paperback are natural recyclable products made from wood grown in sustainable forests. The manufacturing processes conform to the environmental regulations of the country of origin.

Hodder & Stoughton
A Division of Hodder Headline Ltd
338 Euston Road
London NW1 3BH
www.madaboutbooks.com

Contents

Foreword	ix
Acknowledgements	x

1 The importance of strokes

What is stroke?	1
The size of the problem	2
Tackling stroke	3

2 Types of stroke

Factors determining the impact of a stroke	5
Brain cell injury	6
Types of stroke	6
Temporary or permanent damage from stroke	8
Types of transient ischaemic attacks (TIAs)	11
Glossary of other terms for stroke	12

3 The brain and the nervous system

Brain facts	14
Brain structure	15
The 'wiring' of the nervous system	18
The specialised areas of the brain	20
Other specialised areas of the brain	22
Cerebellum	26
Brain stem	26

4 The blood supply to the brain

The main arteries to the brain	29
'Territories' of blood flow	31

5 The symptoms of stroke and transient ischaemic attack (TIA) — 35
Main symptoms — 35
Action in stroke and TIA — 37

6 General treatment for stroke and TIA — 40
Rapid medical assessment — 40
Accurate diagnosis — 43
Brain scans — 43
Artery scans — 44
Other tests — 45
Restore the blood supply if possible — 47
Action to minimise brain injury — 47
Good general care — 50
Difficult decisions — 51
Early stroke care facilities in the UK — 52

7 Treatment for stroke due to artery blockage (ischaemic stroke) — 54
Aspirin — 55
Other anti-platelet drugs — 56
'Clot-dissolving' drugs — 57
Treatment to 'thin the blood' — 59
Carotid artery surgery — 60

8 Treatment for stroke due to artery bleeding (haemorrhagic stroke) — 63
Background information — 63
Aims of treatment — 64
Other surgical aspects of brain haemorrhage — 65
General aspects of treatment — 66

9 Rehabilitation — 68
Mobility and movement — 69
Communication and speech — 73
Intellectual impairment — 75
Body awareness — 76
Nutrition and swallowing — 77
Emotions and relationships — 79
Continence — 81
Work — 82
Driving — 84

10 Stroke risk — 86
Non-modifiable risk factors for stroke — 87
Modifiable risk factors for stroke — 88
Hardening of the arteries – 'atherosclerosis' — 90
How arteries finally become blocked — 91

11 Tackling the main modifiable risk factors for stroke — 94
High blood pressure (hypertension) — 95
How to keep your blood pressure down — 98
Alcohol — 100
Obesity — 101
Exercise — 102
Smoking — 103
Diabetes — 104
Raised blood cholesterol — 106
Atrial fibrillation — 108

12 Information for carers — 111
Help is available — 112
Information helps — 112
Psychological and emotional effects of stroke — 113
Reactions to long-term illness — 114

Look after yourself	115
Take breaks	115
Keep positive	116
Appendix A: References	118
Appendix B: Drugs used in the treatment or prevention of stroke	120
Appendix C: Useful contacts	130

Foreword

Stroke is the third commonest cause of death and the single most important cause of disability in adult life. So it is important that the disease and its implications are fully understood. Recovery after a stroke can be impressive and is aided by many different professionals who work in a multi-disciplinary team in a Stroke Unit. These professionals include doctors, nurses, physiotherapists, occupational therapists, speech and language therapists, dieticians, and most importantly the patients themselves and their friends and relatives. To facilitate this, stroke patients and their carers need access to full information.

Adjustment to disabilities can be difficult and some say life is never quite the same after a stroke. None the less there are strategies available which can help with adjusting to life after a stroke.

This simple to read and easy to use handbook gives stroke patients and their relatives and friends an insight into the disease process and its implications. It details how stroke risk can be reduced by lifestyle changes. It tells how recovery can occur after a stroke. It details in simple terms how primary and secondary prevention, medication which the doctor prescribes, can help prevent a stroke occurring in the future. It gives patients and their loved ones hope. It is a book that every member of the general public should read.

Dr Ron MacWalter
BMSc. (Hons), MD FRCP (Edin), RFCP (Glas)
Consultant Physician and Reader in Medicine
Acute Stroke Unit
Ninewells Hospital & Medical School
Dundee
Scotland

Acknowledgements

I am particularly grateful to Dr Ron MacWalter, Consultant Stroke Physician at Ninewells Hospital and Medical School, Dundee, for reviewing the text. It has been my experience in writing this book series that my busiest colleagues are the ones most willing to find the time from somewhere to help with their production. Stroke medicine is changing fast and Ron has provided the insight of someone expert in his field to keep me on the right track. If any errors still remain in this book it is through no fault of my reviewer.

Cecilia Moore, my editor at Hodder & Stoughton deserves considerable praise not only for assembling the parts into a (hopefully) coherent whole but also for her remarkable patience in dealing with a deadline-averse author.

As always I must thank my wife Anne and son David for giving me the time, space and encouragement to write.

Dr Dan Rutherford
BSc., MB, ChB, MRCGP, FRCP (Edin)

Medical Director
www.netdoctor.co.uk

Chapter 1

The importance of strokes

What is stroke?

'Stroke' is a general term for what happens when a fault develops in the blood supply to a part of the brain. The word 'stroke' implies something that happens suddenly, even dramatically. Often that is exactly what happens: strokes can and do come out of the blue and can strike a person down, including someone who had previously felt perfectly well. 'Brain attack' is another phrase used to mean stroke and it conveys the same sense of suddenness. Not all strokes are, however, so obvious. Sometimes a stroke can be quite subtle and its impact is hard to detect. Most people who have a stroke have only one stroke in their life, but some have multiple strokes.

From the technical point of view we know that there are many different types of strokes. We also know a lot about the causes of strokes, about how to reduce the risk of strokes occurring and about how to best treat strokes when they happen. Information on all of these topics is included in this book. But the effect a stroke has on a person, on their family and on their life in general is a highly individual matter. In a real sense you could say that there are as many different types of stroke as there are people who have strokes.

The size of the problem

In the UK over 150,000 people every year have a stroke. Most people who have a stroke survive it, but, even so, strokes are the third most common cause of death. Many stroke survivors make good recoveries but most are left with at least some degree of permanent disability – currently over a quarter of a million people are in this situation in the UK. Strokes are therefore among the most important of all medical conditions. Although strokes are much more common in older age groups, they do occur in younger people. In the UK 10,000 strokes annually occur in people under the age of 55, and 1000 of these people are under 30. A quarter of all people who have a stroke are of working age.

Compared to heart disease and cancer, stroke has historically tended to have a much lower profile than it deserves. This has been partly due to an incorrect but popular view that not much can be done to prevent strokes happening, and that there is not much that can be done to treat strokes. This view has been widely held among doctors as well as by the public. The attitude used to be that if someone had a stroke then it was a matter of crossing fingers and sitting it out until the condition stabilised and then working at rehabilitation afterwards. This passive attitude has also been reflected in the amount of effort put into researching stroke up to now – it has been said that for every pound spent on stroke research twenty pounds have been spent on heart disease and fifty on cancer.

Tackling stroke

In the past ten years or so it has become increasingly clear that stroke is a condition that needs to be, and can be, tackled more vigorously and that the old 'wait and see' approach is no longer acceptable. We now know that it is possible to help people make a better recovery from stroke when it is treated actively. Furthermore, we also know that an individual's risk of having a stroke is partly dependent on a number of important 'risk factors', many of which can be improved with treatment. Undertaking such treatment lowers that person's future risk of stroke.

For example, having high blood pressure is one of the most important contributing factors to anyone's risk of stroke. Despite the vast amount of medical and scientific knowledge that exists about high blood pressure, and despite the fact that it is a topic about which the public are reasonably aware, it is still a condition that is far from well managed in the general population. The majority of adults with high blood pressure in the UK are either undiagnosed or they are receiving treatment that is insufficient to bring their blood pressure down to safe levels. More effective detection and treatment of this common medical condition would dramatically reduce the numbers of people who have a stroke each year.

Reducing the risk of stroke can be applied both to people who have already had a stroke, and to those who have never had one. In the case of someone who has already had a stroke such action is called 'secondary prevention'. Ideally of course we want to prevent strokes happening in the first place, which is the process called 'primary prevention'. As the example of high blood pressure illustrates, primary and secondary stroke prevention can potentially provide great benefits, but there remains a great deal of work to be done to achieve these results. That work is not exclusively the responsibility of the various health professions. There is much that the individual can do to improve their general fitness and consequently their risk of stroke. We are increasingly seeing the benefits that co-operation between the public and health professionals can bring. A key factor in making that partnership work is greater public knowledge and understanding of the important medical problems that we need to tackle in this day and age. It is now very clear that the lifestyle choices we make can have profound effects on our health. It is also clear that it is never too late to improve our ways. Books such as this are written in the hope of contributing a little to that public understanding.

Stroke is no longer the Cinderella subject it used to be, although it could do with a still higher profile. The UK has lagged significantly behind many other developed countries in the efforts we have put into tackling stroke, but we are beginning to catch up. Stroke is without doubt one of the most important mainstream medical issues that we need to address, especially as older people make up an increasing proportion of our population. There is now much medical research underway to discover more about how the brain responds to injury and how it can be helped to recover. There is every reason to be much more positive about stroke now than we have ever been before.

Key Points

- A stroke is a type of brain damage ('brain attack') caused by impairment of the blood supply to a part of the brain, or leakage of blood into the brain.
- Strokes are among the most common of all major medical illnesses and are the main cause of severe disability in adults.
- Strokes are treatable and the medical management of stroke is now much more active than it used to be.
- A great deal can be done to reduce the chance of a stroke occurring in any individual, by attending to any risk factors the person may have, such as high blood pressure. This also applies to people who have already had a stroke.

Chapter 2

Types of stroke

Factors determining the impact of a stroke

Blood reaches all parts of the body via the complicated network of blood vessels called arteries. The largest artery in the body is the aorta, which starts at the heart. From the aorta large main branches take blood to the limbs, trunk and head. Along the way these arteries divide into progressively smaller ones, much like the branches of a tree. The smallest 'twigs' of this system are blood vessels just a fraction of a millimetre wide.

Strokes are due to some form or other of interruption to the blood supply to the brain – either a blockage to the flow or a leak of blood. Sometimes the interruption is brief, in which case the effects may be fairly short-lived. Brain cells do not withstand the loss of their blood supply for long – just a few minutes is enough to cause a brain cell to die. The amount of *time* for which the blood supply is interrupted is therefore very important in determining the size and impact of a stroke.

The *size* of the artery that gets blocked is another main factor that decides the effects of a stroke. When the artery is a tiny one then the amount of brain tissue affected is correspondingly small. Should the problem occur in one of the larger arteries then a much larger area of brain will be disturbed or damaged. Some very small regions of the brain are extremely important in what they do, so the impact of a small stroke in a critical area can be much greater than its size might suggest. The *location* of a stroke within the brain is the third main detail that decides its impact. The fourth is the *type* of stroke. As we'll see shortly there are two main types – those due to blockage of the brain and those due to bleeding from the brain.

Brain cell injury

Brain cells do not renew themselves when injured in the way that a broken bone or a cut in the skin does. Every part of the brain has a job to do and there are no areas of the brain that are truly redundant or dispensable. In other words, there is probably no such thing as a 'minor stroke'. Yet one of the most extraordinary facts about the human brain is its adaptability. People can and do make remarkable recoveries from strokes that at first are considerably disabling or in which fairly large sections of brain are damaged. A lot depends on just exactly where the damage occurs. In the next chapter some information on the regions of the brain will expand on this topic.

Types of stroke

There are two main ways in which the blood flow in an artery can be stopped from getting through properly. Consequently there are two main types of stroke:

AN ARTERY BECOMES BLOCKED
This can happen in one of two ways:

1. As we get older the internal lining of our arteries gets thicker or 'furred up', so the width of the available channel for blood gets narrower. Eventually the artery can close up altogether. This is what is meant by 'hardening of the arteries'. This is the most common of all types of stroke.
2. A piece of material, such as a blood clot, travels from another part of the circulation and gets jammed in a brain artery, stopping blood from getting through. Usually the source of the clot is the heart itself or an area within one of the main arteries in the neck, for reasons that will be detailed later.

AN ARTERY RUPTURES
Arteries are basically pipes and the blood that flows through them is under pressure. If a weak point in the wall of an artery develops it may eventually give way. Then blood leaks out (haemorrhages) into the surrounding area. That means that blood does not go forward properly to supply the tissues for which it is intended. In the case of an artery leaking deep within the brain the direct physical effects of the leaking blood can damage the surrounding fragile brain tissue. Blood that leaks out of an artery also occupies a space within the fixed volume of the bony skull. That means that healthy brain tissue may become compressed in some types of brain haemorrhage.

Brain aneurysm
In the case of strokes due to rupture of a brain artery, the weak point that eventually gives way may have been present for years beforehand. Some people are probably born with one or more such weak points and others develop them during the course of their life. Typically the weak area is like a bubble on the side of a normal artery. Such a structure is called an aneurysm (*an-yoo-*

rism). The term 'berry aneurysm' is often used because of their resemblance in shape to a small fruit berry on a twig (i.e. the artery). Aneurysms tend to lack the thick muscular wall of a normal artery. Instead they are thin-walled and liable to rupture, especially if the person's blood pressure suddenly goes up for some reason. Unfortunately there is no practical way of diagnosing the presence of a brain aneurysm in most people before it ruptures. Fortunately aneurysms do not always rupture and many of us who have one go through life entirely unaware of and untroubled by its existence.

The two main types of stroke are therefore:

1. Those due to *blockage* of an artery. About 85 per cent of strokes are of this type. Doctors call them *ischaemic* (*is-kee-mik*) strokes. ('Ischaemia' is the medical term for when blood does not get through an artery that is narrowed for any reason.)
2. Those due to *rupture* of an artery. These account for about 15 per cent of strokes. They are technically called *haemorrhagic* (*hem-o-raj-ik*) strokes.

These two types are illustrated in figure 1.

It is not possible for a doctor to tell only by speaking to and examining someone whether their stroke has been due to blockage or rupture of an artery. Specialised tests such as brain scans are needed for that. It is, however, important to distinguish between the two types of stroke, as there are differences in some aspects of their treatment. More detail on these issues will also be presented later.

Temporary or permanent damage from stroke

'TEMPORARY' STROKE

Sometimes the effects of a stroke are short-lived. For example, a tiny clot from some other part of the circulation may jam in a small brain artery, blocking the flow and causing sudden symptoms.

Types of stroke

Figure 1: The main types of stroke

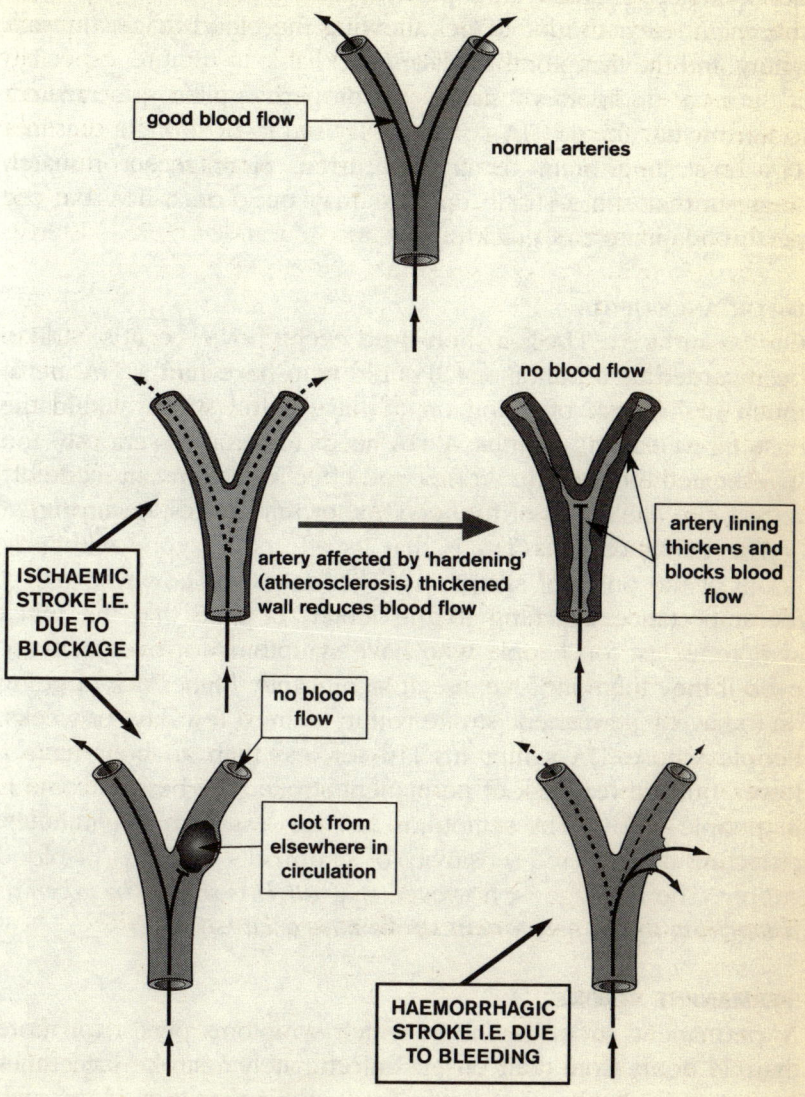

However, within the blood we also have a complicated clot-dissolving system that can cope with small clots. Over a short time this might clear the blockage, allowing the blood to get through again, and the symptoms to disappear.

Such a 'temporary' stroke is properly called a 'transient ischaemic attack', or 'TIA' for short. It used to be thought that in a TIA no lasting brain damage occurred. More recent research suggests that some subtle damage may occur in a TIA but the person adapts to this quickly.

IMPORTANCE OF TIA

On the surface a TIA is a short-lived event; however, it is NOT to be regarded as a minor one. People who have had a TIA are at much higher risk of going on to have a full stroke within the ensuing weeks and months. A TIA needs to be taken seriously and investigated thoroughly. Prompt and effective action can markedly reduce the likelihood of further TIAs, or full strokes, occurring.

The definition of a TIA is that its effects are gone within 24 hours of the onset of symptoms. This does not, however, reflect the importance attaching to the length of time that the initial symptoms last for. People who have symptoms for over an hour, even if they then improve, are at significantly higher risk of going on to have a 'permanent' stroke within the next few days or weeks. People whose TIA symptoms last for less than an hour have a lower, but still real, risk of permanent stroke. The best outcome is in people whose TIA symptoms last for less than ten minutes, reflecting the extreme sensitivity of brain cells to a loss of blood supply. The message is, however, that *all TIAs should be taken as a warning that a permanent stroke may occur soon.*

'PERMANENT' STROKE

A 'permanent' stroke is one in which symptoms persist for more than 24 hours from their onset. Unfortunately a stroke sometimes proves to be fatal within the initial 24-hour time period. In such circumstances it is still, of course, defined as a permanent stroke.

The effects a stroke has may evolve over the course of the first few hours or days, as the level of brain injury settles to its final extent. Doctors often use the term 'completed stroke' to refer to a permanent stroke that has passed this initial state of flux.

Types of transient ischaemic attacks (TIAs)

The basic ways in which a TIA can occur are exactly the same as for any stroke, i.e. due to either *blockage* (ischaemia) or *rupture* (haemorrhage) of an artery. However, a TIA is much more likely to be due to blockage than to rupture. This is because, as in the example above, the blockage may be due to small particles in the blood that break up over a few hours, allowing the blood to flow through again. In the case of a ruptured artery the extra damage to surrounding brain tissue is much less likely to recover quickly, and blood flow to the deprived area is not likely to re-establish itself easily.

Within the first 24 hours it is impossible to tell whether the damage caused by a stroke is going to reverse quickly (i.e. be a TIA) or if it will persist. The immediate medical management of all strokes is therefore the same. It is important to consider a stroke as a medical emergency, requiring prompt investigation and treatment. In chapter 5 we will return to this and review what the symptoms of a stroke or TIA are of which one needs to be aware.

When a stroke happens it can be a bewildering event for all concerned. The brain is such a complicated organ and any form of brain injury can give rise to a vast array of possible effects. Some basic knowledge of the structure of the brain and its blood supply, and some general information on how the brain works, can help to make strokes more understandable. In the next two chapters we will spend some time on this background information.

Glossary of other terms for stroke

Several other words or phrases are often used by health professionals to refer to stroke, and it is as well to know them.

CEREBROVASCULAR ACCIDENT (CVA)

The commonest of these other terms is 'cerebrovascular accident', which is used to cover strokes in general. Usually this is abbreviated to 'CVA'. (It is made up from *cerebro* – meaning 'to do with the brain' and *vascular*, meaning 'to do with the blood vessels'.) At first the word 'accident' seems a bit out of place here. Certainly, no one plans to have a stroke any more than one plans to fall off a ladder! Neither event is entirely predictable, but the more we learn about stroke the more it becomes clear that there is preventive action we can take in advance that reduces our risk of having one. Accidents are similar in some ways. We can reduce but not eliminate their occurrence by taking precautions and thinking ahead.

CEREBRAL THROMBOSIS

A *thrombus* is a clot, and the term cerebral thrombosis if applied correctly means a stroke due to blockage of an artery by the commonest cause, i.e. the 'silting up' process that we also call hardening of the arteries.

CEREBRAL EMBOLISM

An embolism is a particle that travels from one part of the circulation and lands up in another. Such a particle is usually a small clot of blood that has broken free of its source and is floating in the bloodstream. A 'cerebral embolism' therefore means a stroke due to blockage of an artery arising in this way.

TYPES OF BRAIN HAEMORRHAGE

Blood leaking from a ruptured brain artery may travel into the substance of the brain, in which case the terms *cerebral haemorrhage*, or *intracerebral haemorrhage* are commonly used (the prefix *intra* means that it is *within* the brain).

Subarachnoid (*sub-arak-noyd*) haemorrhage refers to bleeding into the space between the brain and the inside of the skull. The subarachnoid space is normally occupied by a clear watery fluid that bathes and cushions the entire brain and spinal cord (cerebrospinal fluid). Subarachnoid haemorrhage is particularly associated with the rupture of a berry aneurysm.

Key Points

- Ischaemic stroke is the commonest type, and is due to blockage of an artery in the brain.
- Artery blockage is usually the end result of 'hardening of the arteries'. The other cause is the lodging of a particle, usually a blood clot that has travelled to the brain from another part of the circulation.
- Haemorrhagic stroke is less common, and is due to rupture of an artery in the brain.
- A stroke becomes defined as such if its effects last more than 24 hours, or if it causes death within 24 hours of onset.
- A transient ischaemic attack (TIA) is exactly the same as a stroke, but apparently complete recovery occurs within 24 hours.
- TIAs are not minor events. The occurrence of a TIA is a warning that a full stroke may be about to occur and it requires prompt action.
- Stroke is a very important medical condition and must be treated urgently. Early treatment of strokes produces better outcomes.
- Cerebrovascular accident, or CVA, is another term that means stroke of any type.

Chapter 3

The brain and the nervous system

Brain facts

The adult human brain weighs, on average, about 1.3kg, or about 2 per cent of an adult's total body weight. The brain, however, consumes eight times more energy than expected on a weight-for-weight basis – 16 per cent of the body's total. The brain demands a constant supply of oxygen and 'fuel' from the bloodstream – significant interruption of blood flow to the brain causes unconsciousness within a few seconds and at normal body temperature brain cells cannot survive more than about three minutes without oxygen. Brain cells use glucose (sugar) almost exclusively for their fuel supply, unlike most other tissues of the body that can also use fats for energy. At any one point in time brain cells store only about 2 minutes' worth of glucose, so they need constantly to top this up from the bloodstream. It is therefore easy to see why any interruption to the blood supply of the brain causes almost immediate effects.

Unlike many other types of cell in the body, brain cells are not replaced when they die. If an area of brain is completely starved of blood for long enough – just a few minutes – then those brain cells are lost forever. How the brain adapts to injury despite the loss of brain tissue is not well understood, but it seems that tasks that used to be carried out by the injured area of the brain can sometimes be taken over by other, healthy parts of the brain. Not all functions of the brain are capable of being relocated in this way. Vision, for example, if lost through stroke injury can not be regained, but other functions such as power loss can sometimes be built up again by practice and retraining. The recovery may not be complete but it can be enough to regain independence in the action lost.

Brain structure

Figure 2 shows the general structure of the brain. The right and left halves ('hemispheres') are extensively interconnected by nerve fibres (the 'white matter') that relay messages to and from different parts of the brain and, via the spinal cord, every part of the body. The surface layer of each hemisphere of the brain (the 'grey matter') is folded and made up mainly of nerve cells, called neurones.

There are over 100 billion neurones in the brain and nervous system of a human being, each only a few thousandths of a millimetre across. An individual neurone is shown in diagrammatic form in figure 3, magnified many thousands of times. A single main nerve fibre arises from the cell body and it conducts the main signals originating from a particular neurone. This fibre divides into many smaller branches, which in turn eventually make contact with other neurones. Each neurone also receives signals from other neurones through fibres connected to its cell body. The network of connections between nerve cells is enormously complex – there are said to be more possible ways for the

Figure 2: The brain

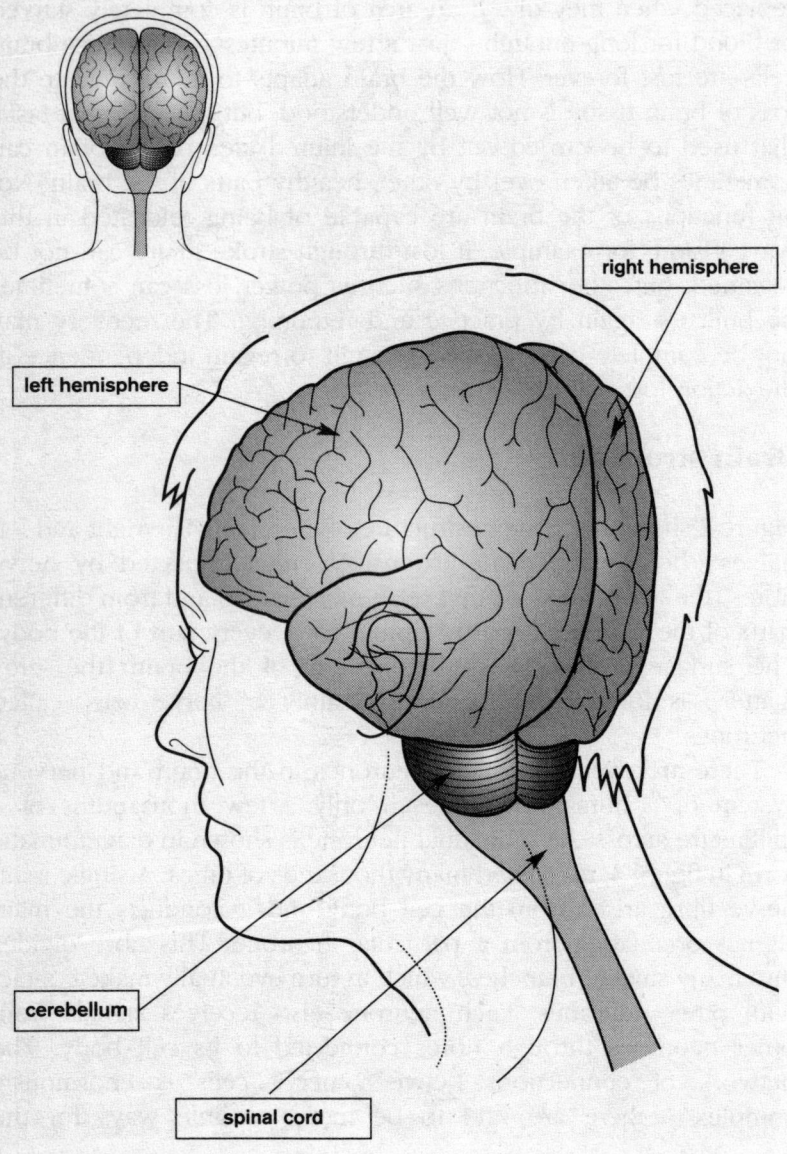

The brain and the nervous system

Figure 3: Nerve cell ('Neurone')

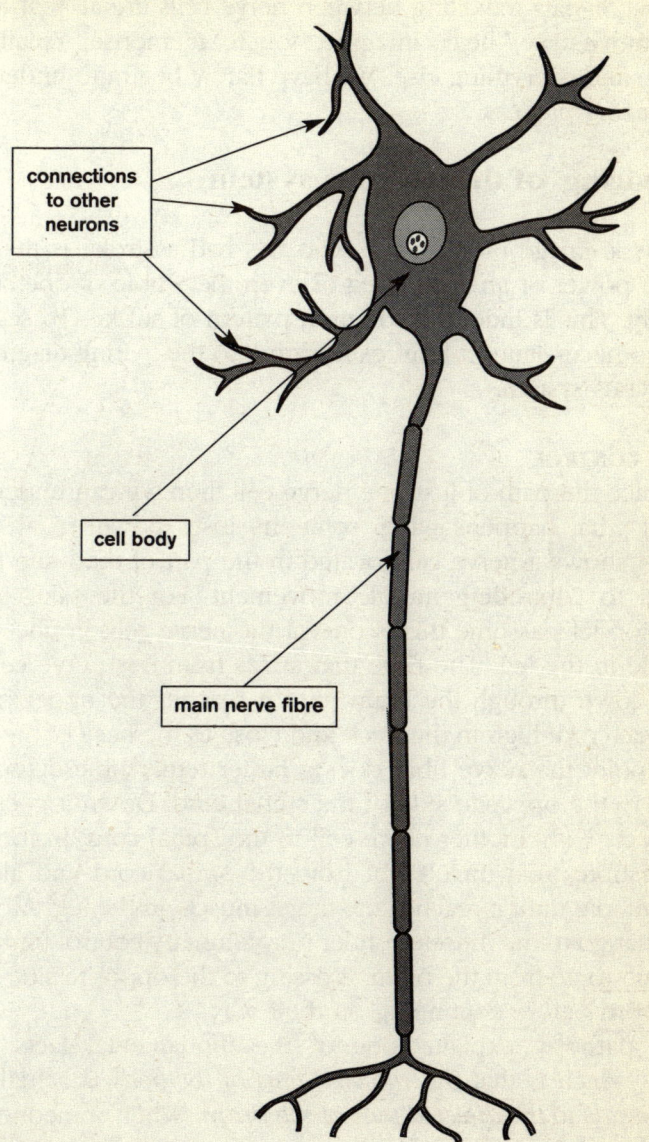

17

neurones in one person to link up than there are atoms in the Universe! Signals travelling between nerve cells are all that lets us think, move, see, hear, imagine, touch, memorise, recall, feel emotion and everything else. We have barely begun to understand this amazing process.

The 'wiring' of the nervous system

The classic image of someone who has had a stroke is that they lose the power of an arm, a leg or even the whole of one side of the body. This is indeed a common pattern of stroke. To see why this is so necessitates a brief excursion into the 'wiring diagram' of the nervous system.

MUSCLE CONTROL

If we trace the path of just one nerve cell then we can understand most of what happens when someone loses power in a stroke. Figure 4 shows a nerve cell located in the part of the brain that is devoted to controlling muscle movement. For the sake of this illustration let's assume this is one of the nerve cells connected to a muscle in the leg. The fibre that arises from this nerve cell first travels down through the brain until it reaches the upper part of the spinal cord, high in the neck and close to the base of the skull. At this point the nerve fibre does a rather remarkable detour and crosses to the opposite side of the spinal cord. Down it goes until it connects with another nerve cell in the spinal cord, from which a nerve fibre then travels out from the spinal cord and along a nerve bundle until it reaches the target muscle in the leg. All nerve fibres that go to the muscles under our voluntary control undertake this same route from the brain, crossing to the opposite side of the spinal cord before continuing on their way.

This pathway explains one of the fundamental facts about strokes, which is that the *affected part of the body* is actually the *opposite side to the affected part of the brain*. When someone loses

The brain and the nervous system

Figure 4: Path of a 'motor nerve' (i.e. a nerve to a muscle)

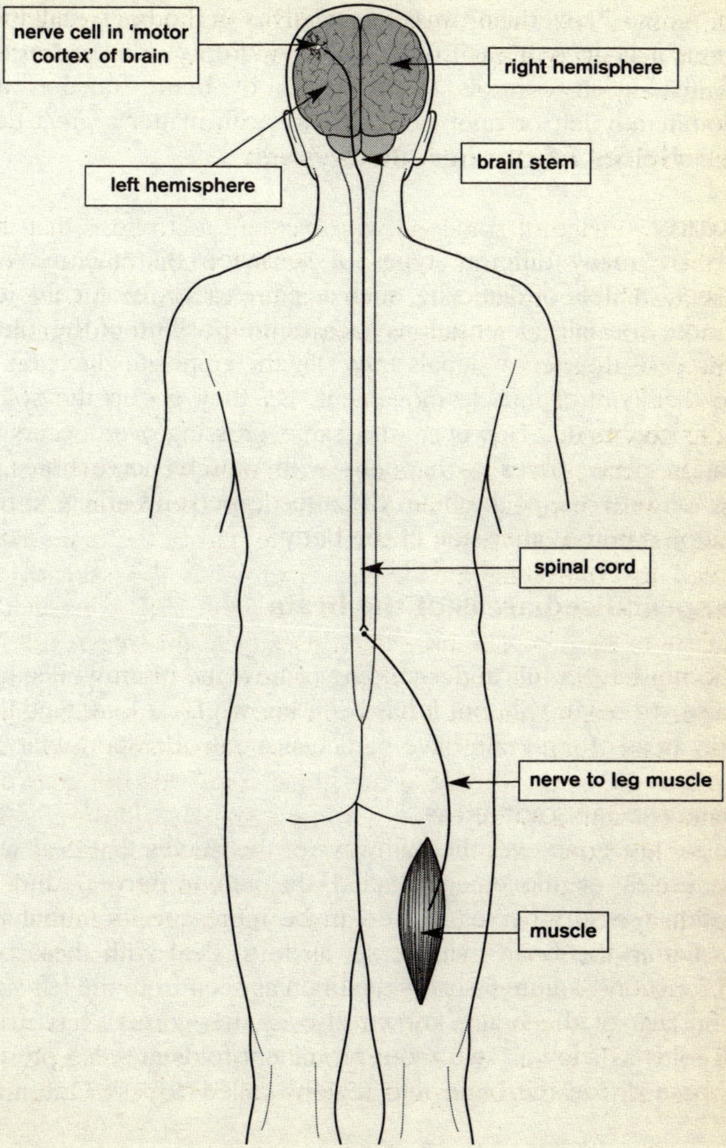

- nerve cell in 'motor cortex' of brain
- right hemisphere
- left hemisphere
- brain stem
- spinal cord
- nerve to leg muscle
- muscle

power on their right side it is because they have had a blockage or leakage of an artery on the left side of their brain, and vice versa. As we'll cover shortly, the two halves of the brain may look like mirror images of each other but they are not identical in the tasks that each controls. Some types of brain function are predominantly left or right sided. Thus it can matter a great deal on which side of the brain a stroke occurs.

SENSATION

There are many different types of sensation that the nervous system is capable of detecting, such as pain, touch, heat, cold, itch and more specialised sensations such as the position of the joints. In this case the nerve signals travel in the opposite direction to those that control muscle movement, i.e. they go up the spinal cord to the brain. However, the same crossing-over occurs of sensation nerve fibres as happens with muscle nerve fibres. A stroke on one side of the brain can affect a person's ability to feel sensations on the other side of the body.

The specialised areas of the brain

We do not have a full understanding of how the brain works, and perhaps we never will, but it has been known for a long time that certain areas of the brain have particular areas of responsibility.

'MOTOR' AND 'SENSORY' AREAS

We have just gone over the pathways of the nerves that deal with the muscles of movement (called the *motor* nerves) and of sensation (*sensory* nerves). One can be more specific about the areas within the brain that are set aside to deal with these two main functions. Figure 5 shows the brain as seen from the left side. The surface of the brain, known also as the 'cortex', has many small folds as shown. Two more prominent folds are also present and these divide the brain into regions called 'lobes'. One main

The brain and the nervous system

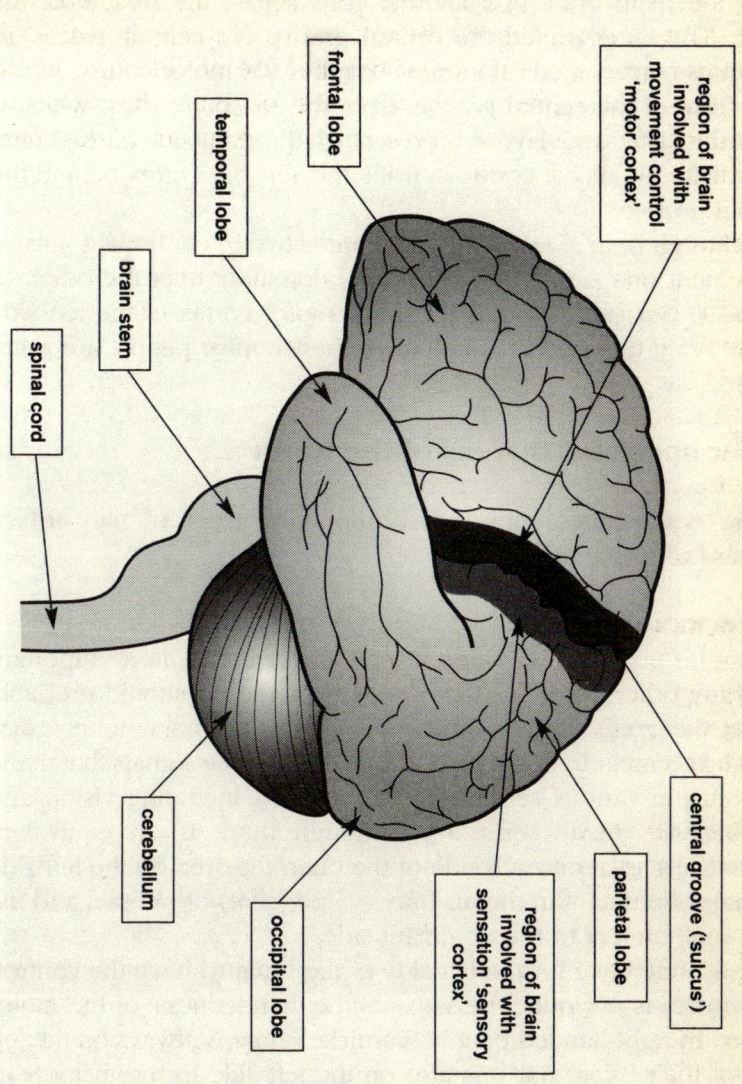

Figure 5: 'Motor' and 'sensory' areas of the brain

21

fold divides the side part of the brain, called the temporal lobe, from the main brain and another runs across the middle of the brain. The latter, called the central groove (or central 'sulcus' to give it its correct medical name) separates the motor cortex, which is in front of the central groove, from the sensory cortex, which is behind it. The same layout is present on the right side of the brain, again with the motor cortex in front and sensory cortex behind the central groove.

Although both sides of the brain are active in controlling muscle movement one side tends to become dominant over the other. In about 90 per cent of people it is the motor cortex of the left side of the brain that becomes dominant, hence most people are right-handed.

Other specialised areas of the brain

Figure 6 illustrates some other important areas of the surface (cortex) of the brain.

WERNICKE'S AREA

It may be unfair to rank any part of the brain as more important than any other but if such an award is merited it should probably go to the zone in the upper part of the temporal lobe called Wernicke's area. In this region of the brain all the signals that come in from the various sensations of the body, including vision and hearing, are made sense of. Although there is an equivalent 'Wernicke's area' on each side of the brain the area on the left side becomes dominant in the majority (95 per cent) of people, and the term really refers to the dominant side.

This preference for the left side of the brain to have the controlling power is not quite the same as the 'handedness' of the motor cortex. In right-handed people Wernicke's area is always on the left side of their brain, but it is also on the left side in the majority of left-handed people (in whom their right motor cortex is dominant).

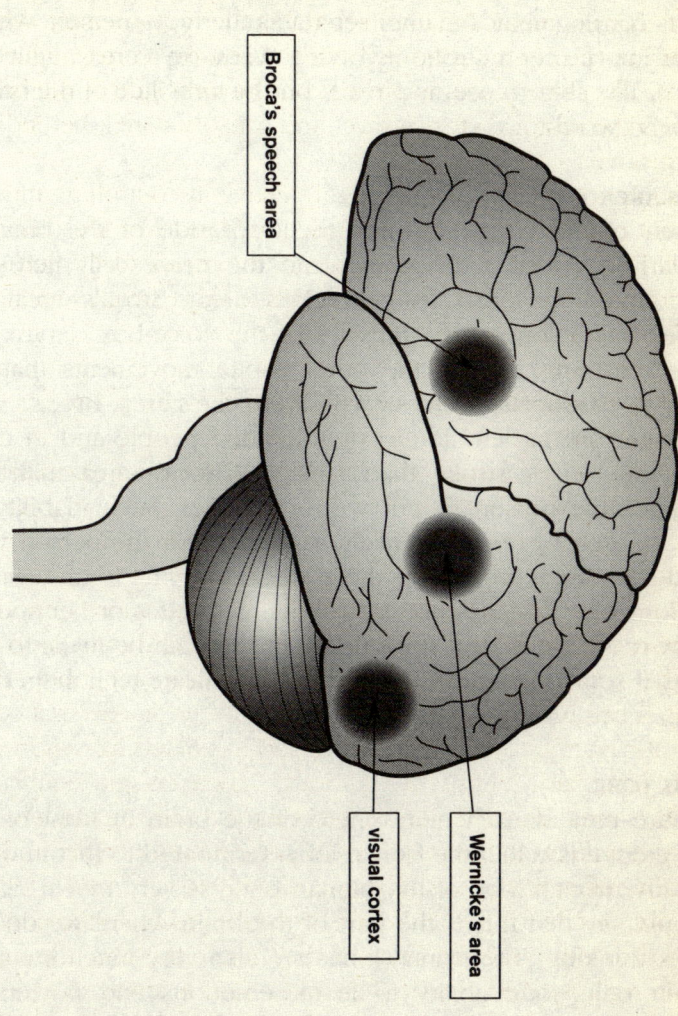

Figure 6: Other specialised areas of the brain

Damage to Wernicke's area affects a person's ability to make sense of the input he or she receives from the senses. In particular it makes it hard for that person to understand speech, despite the fact that hearing may be unaffected. Similarly, a person whose vision is intact after a stroke involving Wernicke's area might still be physically able to see and read, but be unable to understand the printed words.

BROCA'S AREA

This area of the cortex towards the front side of the brain is particularly involved with speech and the nerve cells here are closely linked to those in Wernicke's area. Broca's area co-ordinates the actions of the muscles of the voice-box (larynx) as well as breathing and all the other subtle movements that go together to produce speech. As with Wernicke's area, Broca's area is dominant on the left side in right-handed people and in most left-handers too. A stroke that damages Broca's area makes it difficult for the person to put words together. Such inability to express oneself can be immensely frustrating for the person who has had a stroke as well as for those who are trying to understand them. Someone who has had a stroke affecting his or her speech in this way is neither deaf nor stupid but they can be made to feel that way if someone who is trying to communicate with them does not appreciate what the problem is.

FRONTAL LOBE

The entire part of each hemisphere of the brain in front of the central groove is called the frontal lobe. Compared to that in other species the frontal lobe of the human brain is very much bigger. You could say that this is the part of the brain where we do our complex thinking. The frontal lobes are also very much involved with our behaviour, ability to learn, emotions and powers of judgement. Disorders of any or all of these functions can occur in someone who has a stroke in a frontal lobe. Unlike the motor cortex or Wernicke's and Broca's areas no one frontal lobe seems to become dominant over the other. Instead, the frontal lobes work in collaboration with each other, via the enormous number of connecting nerves that run from side to side deeper in the brain.

The effects of frontal lobe damage are much harder to predict than for damage to the more specialised areas such as Broca's speech area. Quite substantial damage to the frontal lobes can on occasion give rise to hardly any problems. Frontal lobe damage, when apparent, can cause a loss of the ability to plan actions or it can cause someone's personality to change. Typically, they may become indifferent to events around them or may become unpredictable and liable to shoot off at a tangent any time.

PARIETAL LOBE

The zone behind the central groove that extends nearly to the back of the brain is called the parietal (*par-eye-et-al*) lobe. The actions of this part of the brain make us aware of where we are in space and how we relate to our surroundings and to other parts of our own body. Damage to a parietal lobe may cause a person to neglect the opposite side of their body (i.e. the same side as the paralysis). For example, someone may fail to recognise that his arm, now paralysed from a stroke, is actually part of his own body at all. He may also ignore stimuli, including vision, coming in from the side opposite to the brain damage, even although physically he can still see and feel sensations normally.

OCCIPITAL LOBE

The 'occiput' (*ok-si-poot*) is the back of the head and it is at the back of the brain that nerve fibres from the eyes finally deliver their signals. The pathway that nerve fibres from the eyes take on their way back through the skull is just as complex as those of the spinal cord nerve fibres that cross to the opposite side. Without going into unnecessary detail, each eye sends half of its nerve fibres to the same side and half to the other side of the brain. A stroke that damages the occipital lobe of the brain may cause blindness, or partial blindness, despite the fact that the eyes are undamaged.

Cerebellum

Figure 6 also shows an area at the back of the brain, which looks rather different to the main part of the brain. This is the 'cerebellum', which literally means 'little brain'. The cerebellum is richly connected to other parts of the brain, notably the motor cortex, and it also receives a great deal of information from sensation nerves in the muscles, tendons and joints all over the body. The main function of the cerebellum is to co-ordinate the movements of the muscles of the body – almost all movements require many different muscles to be made to work together in smooth co-operation.

If part of the cerebellum is affected by a stroke the typical effects are seen in the person's balance and co-ordination. They may become quite unsteady on their feet and prone to falls, or develop difficulty with moving their hands or limbs in a co-ordinated way. Previously familiar tasks can then become much more difficult to perform. Damage to the cerebellum does not cause paralysis of the muscles, but instead causes a loss of their control.

Brain stem

Again referring back to figure 6, the last, but not least, part of this tour of the brain is the brain stem. This is the area at the top of the spinal cord at the junction between the spinal cord and the brain. Every nerve that travels between the brain and the spinal cord has to go through the brain stem, so it's first importance is as a main trunk route, densely packed with the nerves controlling our muscles and relaying sensations. Additionally however, the brain stem contains within it many of the 'control centres' that regulate various body functions. For example, within the brain stem are special nerve cells that control our breathing, pulse rate, blood pressure and digestive system. Also in the brain stem are nerves that control the movements of the eye muscles and yet others that are essential to our sense of balance. Motor and sensation nerves for the face and head are also located in the brain stem, including those that control movements of the tongue.

Many important structures are therefore packed into the small space of the brain stem and a stroke here can have a major impact. For example, if the control centre for breathing is affected this could rapidly prove fatal. Other possible effects of a brain stem stroke are loss of balance, double vision, impaired swallowing or other problems with movements of the muscles of the face or of sensations from the face.

Key Points

- Brain cells require a continuous supply of blood to provide them with oxygen and glucose. Brief interruption of the blood supply to the brain causes almost immediate effects.
- When brain cells are damaged new brain cells are not made to replace them. However, the lost function can sometimes be undertaken by other, healthy parts of the brain.
- The nerves that control muscles or convey sensations such as touch cross to the opposite side of the body en route to and from the brain. The physical effects of a stroke are therefore usually seen on the side of the body opposite to the area of damaged brain.
- The left side of the brain tends to be dominant in the interpretation of information from the senses (Wernicke's area) and in the control of speech (Broca's area).

- The frontal lobes of the brain are the areas where we do our most complex thinking. Damage to the frontal lobes can affect a person's personality, their ability to think clearly, their emotional state and their judgement, among other things.
- The parietal lobes at the side of the brain make sense of where we are in space, including with respect to our own body.
- The occipital lobes at the back of the brain are where vision is perceived. A stroke here can cause partial or full loss of sight.
- The cerebellum is the area at the back of the brain that is crucial to co-ordinating muscle movements.
- The brain stem contains many of the important control centres for automatic body functions such as breathing, pulse and blood pressure. It also has important roles in the control of balance and of movements of the eyes and the face.

Chapter 4

The blood supply to the brain

A little more detail on the blood supply to the brain helps in understanding the patterns of disability commonly seen as a result of a stroke.

The main arteries to the brain

Figure 7 shows the basic details of the four main arteries that supply blood to the brain.

CAROTID ARTERIES
The two large arteries that run up either side of the neck are the *carotid* arteries. At about the angle of the jaw each main carotid artery divides into two, sending a deeper branch in to serve the brain. These are called the *internal carotid* arteries and together they make up the 'carotid system' of the brain's blood supply.

Figure 7: Blood supply to the brain

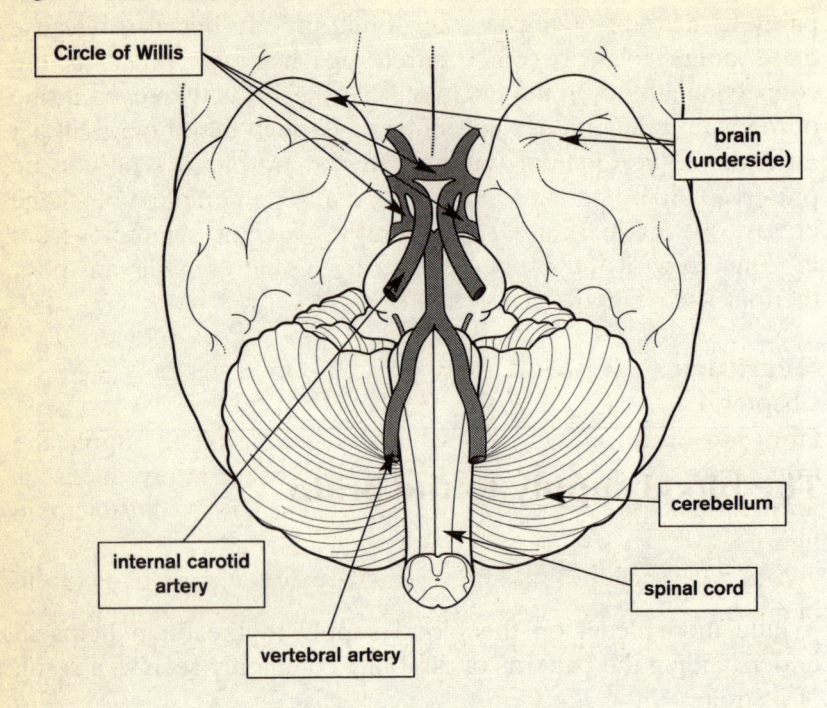

Labels: Circle of Willis; brain (underside); cerebellum; spinal cord; vertebral artery; internal carotid artery

VERTEBROBASILAR ARTERIES
The two other main arteries that supply the brain run up through holes in the bones (vertebrae) of the neck. Each of these is called a *vertebral* artery. Each vertebral artery then joins with the other to form a single artery called the *basilar* artery. The combination of these arteries is known as the 'vertebrobasilar system'.

CIRCLE OF WILLIS
Smaller arteries link between the internal carotid and the basilar arteries at the base of the brain, sharing the blood flow between the two systems. This produces what is nearly a ring-shaped arrangement of arteries called the *Circle of Willis*. Just how wide

each of these connecting arteries is varies between individuals, partly as a result of how we are built anyway but also because these arteries can become 'furred up' like any other. If the connecting arteries in the Circle of Willis are wide then even if one of the main brain arteries gets blocked enough blood may still get through via the Circle of Willis for the brain's blood supply to be preserved. Some people can therefore suffer a complete blockage of, say, one internal carotid artery and yet have no symptoms from it. Conversely, if the connections in the Circle of Willis are poor then no such 'failsafe' action will occur.

'Territories' of blood flow

From the Circle of Willis further arteries come off to supply the front and the middle of the brain. The basilar artery sends its further branches to the back of the brain. This is illustrated in figure 8.

You will recall from the previous chapter that some parts of the brain have specific functions, and if that information is now combined with knowledge of the brain's blood supply then one can predict to some extent what sort of patterns of stroke are likely to be seen.

CAROTID TERRITORY

The carotid territory of the middle and front parts of the brain includes the motor cortex, the sensory cortex, the speech area (Broca's), Wernicke's area and the parietal lobes. Strokes arising from the carotid system will therefore tend to cause power loss, abnormal sensations, neglect of the affected side and word-finding difficulties (if the dominant hemisphere is affected). One small but important detail concerning the carotid system is that the blood supply to the eyes arises from these arteries. A condition exists in which tiny particles of blood clot coming from 'upstream' in the arteries get temporarily lodged in the arteries of the eye. This can

Figure 8: 'Territories' of blood supply to the brain

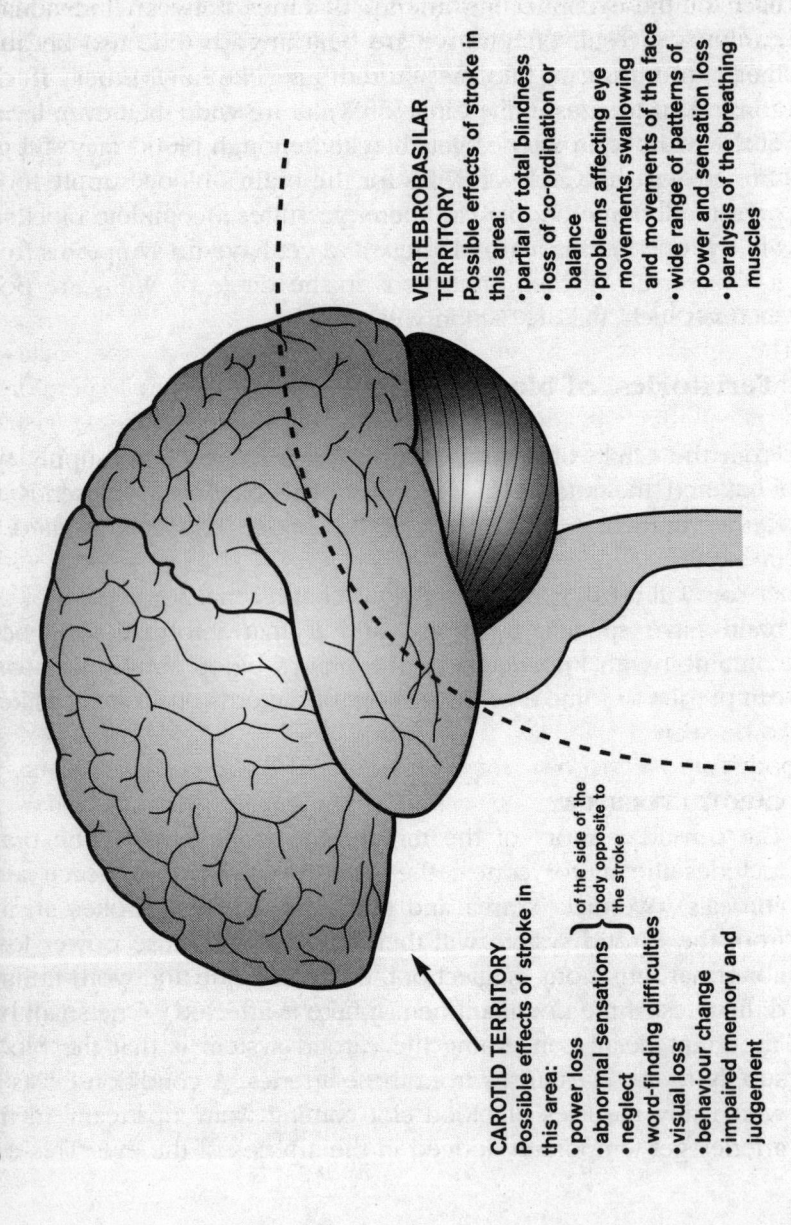

CAROTID TERRITORY
Possible effects of stroke in this area:
- power loss
- abnormal sensations } of the side of the body opposite to the stroke
- neglect
- word-finding difficulties
- visual loss
- behaviour change
- impaired memory and judgement

VERTEBROBASILAR TERRITORY
Possible effects of stroke in this area:
- partial or total blindness
- loss of co-ordination or balance
- problems affecting eye movements, swallowing and movements of the face
- wide range of patterns of power and sensation loss
- paralysis of the breathing muscles

cause temporary loss of vision, or partial loss of vision. If someone develops such a symptom it's a warning that there may be significant furring up of the carotid arteries, and action may need to be taken to stave off the possibility of a stroke occurring later. (This temporary loss of eyesight is therefore a particular type of TIA. Should the flow of blood through an eye artery be permanently blocked this will cause permanent blindness of that eye, which is therefore a particular type of stroke.)

VERTEBROBASILAR TERRITORY

The vertebrobasilar system supplies blood mainly to the back of the brain (occipital lobe), cerebellum and brain stem. Therefore, strokes affecting the vertebrobasilar system may cause visual problems such as partial or total blindness, impaired co-ordination or balance, difficulties with eye movements or swallowing or facial muscle paralysis. Loss of power or of sensation can also occur with a vertebrobasilar stroke because the brain stem is so packed with nerves of all types. As it is in the brain stem that much of the crossing-over of nerve fibres to the opposite side of the body occurs one can also see patterns of power and sensation loss that are not seen in strokes involving the carotid territory. For example, it would be possible in a brain stem stroke for both sides of the body to be affected by the same stroke, if it happened to occur in one of the crossing-over zones. So many combinations of symptoms are possible that it would become confusing to go further than this. The point is that some combinations of disability often go together in stroke, and these can be understood by considering which artery has been involved.

Further 'downstream' from the Circle of Willis there is little or no interconnection between adjacent territories of blood supply. This is one of the basic reasons why strokes occur in the first place: there is little or no chance of blood finding a different route through when one of these deeper brain arteries becomes blocked or bleeds. Another consequence of this way in which the brain's blood supply is arranged is a rare type of stroke called a 'watershed infarct'. This can occur if someone's blood pressure drops and remains very low for enough time. In this case the stroke is due to the failure of enough blood to get out to the furthest reaches of an artery's territory because there is insufficient pressure to get it there.

Key Points

- Four main arteries supply the brain with blood.
- The two carotid arteries run through the sides of the neck.
- The two vertebral arteries run through the vertebrae of the neck before forming the single basilar artery.
- All the arteries are connected at the base of the brain, to a variable degree, in the Circle of Willis.
- Carotid territory strokes are the commonest and are the usual cause of strokes in which one-sided paralysis and loss of sensation or problems with speech and expression are found.
- Vertebrobasilar strokes are more likely to cause permanent visual problems or problems with balance, co-ordination and swallowing.

Chapter 5

The symptoms of stroke and TIA

Main symptoms

Although many of the underlying changes in the body that eventually lead to stroke, such as hardening of the arteries, take years to develop, the most characteristic feature of a stroke or a TIA is that it occurs suddenly. The sudden occurrence of any of the following symptoms could possibly be due to a stroke or a TIA:

Table 1: Main symptoms of stroke or transient ischaemic attack

• Loss of power in an arm, leg or side of the face
• Numbness or tingling in an arm, leg or side of the face
• Slurring or an inability to speak
• Difficulty in understanding language
• Blurring or loss of vision in one or both eyes
• Loss of balance or co-ordination (accompanied by other symptoms)
• Unexplained severe headache (see below)

None of these symptoms is unique to stroke or TIA, and they all have different possible causes. Those at the top of the list, the loss of power or sensation, especially involving only one side of the body, are more strongly associated with stroke.

Those at the bottom – loss of balance and, especially, headache – have a wide range of possible causes. In fact, stroke is only rarely associated with headache. It is included in the list because subarachnoid haemorrhage can cause a severe pain at the back of the head (often called a 'thunderclap' headache because of its suddenness and intensity) and needs to be diagnosed as accurately and as urgently as a stroke. Subarachnoid haemorrhage is, however, a rare condition and usually accompanied by other significant symptoms such as vomiting or even unconsciousness.

Similarly a GP will quite often see patients whose balance has gone off a bit and yet most of those people will not have had a stroke either.

COMBINATIONS OF SYMPTOMS

Although it's quite possible for a stroke to show just one of these main symptoms it's commoner to see more than one at the same time. Armed with the information about the brain's blood supply from the last chapter, you will appreciate how, for example, loss of power in the right arm or leg might occur along with difficulty in speaking, as the 'speech cortex' (Broca's area) and the 'motor cortex' are both served by the carotid artery and its branches.

Other more general symptoms may accompany the early stages of a stroke, such as drowsiness. Often the exact pattern of disability that a stroke causes will alter over the first few hours or days, during which time experts may refer to the stroke 'evolving'.

MULTIPLE SMALL STROKES

Stroke and TIA don't always call such direct attention to themselves as the symptom list above suggests. For example, a problem seen, usually in older people is the effect on general mental function of successive very small strokes. This can lead to dementia (so-called 'vascular dementia'). Although some people with vascular dementia may also have had an obvious stroke or TIA in their history, leading to one of the major disabilities such as power loss in a limb, many others have not. Most people who have a stroke do not, however, develop dementia.

Action in stroke and TIA

The important issue is to remember that stoke and TIA are medical emergencies. The correct action for a medical emergency is to dial 999 and request an ambulance. Delay in calling for emergency medical help in stroke, or suspected stroke, is a continuing problem. At the time of writing of this book (2005) one of the UK's main stroke-related charities, The Stroke Association, has embarked upon a campaign to encourage greater public awareness of the need to act quickly. One part of the campaign is to promote the use of the 'Face, Arm, Speech Test' (FAST), as used by ambulance personnel. It is quick and easy to do and is reproduced in Table 2.

Table 2: Face, Arm, Speech Test – FAST – for suspected stroke or TIA

F	Facial weakness	Can the person smile? Has their mouth or eye drooped?
A	Arm weakness	Can the person raise both arms?
S	Speech problems	Can the person speak clearly and understand what you say?
T	Test all three symptoms	
Any one of the three symptoms is enough reason to suspect a stroke. **The correct action is to dial 999**		

When a stroke reveals itself through the sudden appearance of one of the 'classic' symptoms listed in tables 1 and 2 it should be quite easily recognised. Real life is of course that little bit more complicated! Stroke is not always so clear-cut. The symptoms might be more vague and surveys show that people don't like to 'bother the doctor', especially at night or at the weekend. Remember though that:

- You are not expected to be a doctor or make an accurate diagnosis on yourself or anyone else.
- If it turns out that the symptoms are due to some other less serious cause, then well and good, but that takes time to discover.
- 'Time is brain'. The quicker you act the better.

Remember that TIAs often occur in advance of a full stroke in someone whose risk of stroke can be brought down. The 'window of opportunity' immediately after a TIA should not be missed.

Early action may also limit the damage in permanent stroke. We need to get away from the still-too-common situation in which people with stroke or TIA delay seeking help for days or weeks, by which time little or nothing can be done to alter the outcome.

Key Points

- The main symptoms of stroke and TIA are:
    Loss of power in an arm, leg or side of the face
    Numbness or tingling in an arm, leg or side of the face
    Slurring or an inability to speak
    Difficulty in understanding language
    Blurring or loss of vision in one or both eyes
    Loss of balance or co-ordination.

- Unexplained severe headache is not a symptom of stroke or TIA but may be a symptom of subarachnoid haemorrhage, in which it is usually accompanied by other symptoms.
- The Face, Arm, Speech Test (FAST) is a quick and easy way to assess suspected stroke or TIA.
- Should stroke or TIA be suspected, call for urgent medical attention right away by dialling 999.

Chapter 6

General treatment for stroke and TIA

The basic principles of the early treatment of stroke and TIA are the same:

1. Rapid medical assessment
2. Accurate diagnosis
3. Re-establish the blood supply if possible (in cases of stroke due to artery blockage)
4. Minimise brain injury
5. Good general care

1. Rapid medical assessment

The need for urgent medical attention has been emphasised in the last chapter – we need to get used to treating brain attacks as urgently as we do heart attacks. The first step in the process is that the general public should recognise the signs of stroke and TIA and act on these right away. The second step is that the organised medical services should respond swiftly.

Over the past few years there have been numerous public information drives to make sure we all know that when someone suddenly gets chest pain we don't waste any time before dialling 999. Even so, many people with a heart attack still wait too long before seeing a doctor. If the message about urgency is yet to get through properly in the case of heart attacks, which have had so much attention for decades, it's no great surprise that it will be some time yet before strokes get the same level of priority. However, now that you have read this far you will know what to look for and should have no hesitation in calling for help if you suspect a stroke.

The National Clinical Guidelines for Stroke, published by the Royal College of Physicians of London, contain straightforward recommendations for stroke care:

- Stroke services should be organised so that patients are admitted under the care of a specialist team for their acute care and rehabilitation.
- Any patient with persistent stroke symptoms should be rapidly admitted to hospital, preferably to a stroke unit with the appropriate equipment and training.

Although it does not automatically follow that people with stroke admitted to non-specialist units are getting less than ideal care, statistics show rather starkly that they often do. Survival of people with stroke on a specialist unit is up to 25 per cent better than on a general medical ward. Until we have the ideal situation in place, in which everyone with a stroke is managed by a specialist in the condition, we'll have to compromise and ensure that as far as possible the important elements of good stroke care, as mentioned throughout this book, are applied no matter where the person is cared for.

NON-HOSPITAL CARE

Current recommendations for stroke are that it is hospital-based, i.e. the patient is admitted to hospital. In hospital the best attention can be given to monitoring the person's condition, treating any adverse changes that occur, giving good nursing care and so on. It is much harder to do all of that at home. Quick access to tests such as brain scanning (see next section) is also more easily achieved and often is only practicable if the person is an in-patient. It is, however, not impossible for stroke care to be provided at home. The necessary tests could be done as an out-patient and this may be quite satisfactory in some circumstances, provided all the right sorts of additional assessment and care were carried out. Alternatively, in someone with a number of other disabilities who then had a stroke, it might not be in their best interests to be admitted to an acute hospital, in which case home would be more appropriate.

Given that there should be room for personal choice (which is not as available as it should be in the resource-strapped NHS), current medical evidence shows that the best results in stroke care are achieved when people are admitted to hospital in the early stage of the illness.

ACTION IN RAPIDLY RECOVERING TIA

In the initial stage of stroke or TIA both conditions look the same. TIA improves within 24 hours and often very much quicker – within minutes. Admission to hospital of everyone with the slightest possibility of having had a brief TIA might seem impractical – we don't have the capacity to do this in the NHS. For people who have what seems to be a TIA but whose symptoms clear quickly a compromise is needed, in the form of a rapid access outpatient service that provides the GP with the necessary back-up and advice. In addition, the patient should be fast-tracked through all the necessary investigations. An adequate service ought to be able to see a newly referred patient and complete all such investigations within 14 days. At present (2005) only slightly more than half of hospitals in England, Wales and Northern Ireland can actually provide a service within 14 days. Scotland has not audited its services in the way the rest of the UK has and possibly even fewer hospitals there can deliver this level of service.

2. Accurate diagnosis

Stroke diagnosis is not always straightforward – medical conditions other than stroke can share similar symptoms. Even when it appears very likely that stroke is the diagnosis it is important to distinguish strokes due to artery blockage (ischaemic) from those due to artery leakage (haemorrhagic), as this makes a great deal of difference to the treatment. A person's memory of what happened, and the observations of others, is particularly helpful in assessing TIA, as very often the physical symptoms of a TIA are gone by the time the doctor sees the patient.

We said earlier that a doctor is not able to distinguish between the types of stroke only on the basis of speaking to the patient and making a clinical examination. A brain scan is the only way to make a precise diagnosis. Everyone who has a stroke ought to have a brain scan within 48 hours of the onset of symptoms so that the type of stroke is established. There are two main types of brain scan in common use.

BRAIN SCANS

CT scan
CT is short for 'computerised tomography' and it is a sophisticated type of X-ray. A beam of X-rays is shone through the part of the body being investigated and is picked up by a detector on the far side of the patient. The beam and detector are then rotated through a full circle and a computer then analyses the amount of X-ray that has been able to pass through from every direction.

Using that information the computer can build up an image like a slice through the body at that level. A CT scanner looks like a large ring, through which you slide while lying on a moveable table. It takes only a few minutes to do a CT scan of the brain.

MRI scan

MRI stands for 'magnetic resonance image'. Instead of X-rays MRI scanners use high frequency radio waves to make water molecules in body tissues 'vibrate'. This vibration in turn sets off radio waves from the tissues that the scanner can detect. MRI scanners are similar in appearance to CT scanners in that they comprise a large ring-shaped detector within which the person lies for the duration of the scan. MRI tends to be noisier than CT and takes a lot longer.

There are minor technical differences in the usefulness of the two types of scan but in practical terms both are adequate at sorting strokes into those due to artery blockage and those due to bleeding. In addition to showing the type of stroke, the scan also shows the region of the brain affected.

ARTERY SCANS

In all people with a TIA or stroke involving the carotid arteries further investigation is needed to examine the arteries in detail, looking for a possible area of blockage or source of clots. Although it is possible to extend the use of CT and MRI scans to examine the arteries the commonest way for this test to be done is with ultrasound.

This is a similar technique to that which is commonly used to look at the baby in the womb. High-frequency sound waves are sent from a probe placed against the skin to the structures below. The sound waves bounce back and are detected by the probe, and the attached electronics builds up an image of the tissues below the skin. Ultrasound is good at outlining body structures that contain fluid, so the blood-filled arteries show up well. Ultrasound can also measure the speed of flow of blood through the arteries, so it can detect both the physical narrowing that might be present in an artery as well as the slowing up of the blood flow that such an obstruction causes.

The importance of artery scanning is to pick up those people with narrowing of a carotid artery who would benefit from early surgery to remove the narrowed segment. This topic is dealt with in chapter 7.

Ultrasound is also useful for examining the valves and chambers of the heart. In some people with stroke the heart is the source of tiny clots that are shed and land up in the circulation of the brain. Possible causes of this include damage to the heart valves, perhaps from previous infection, or a recent heart attack, with a clot forming over the damaged muscle within the heart. Ultrasound can outline the structure of the heart very well and will show up any irregularities of the valves or clots inside the heart. Ultrasound scanning of the heart is called echocardiography.

OTHER TESTS

Many other tests are medically useful in assessing a person in the early stages of a stroke or TIA.

Blood pressure

Taking a person's blood pressure is the commonest medical test of all. A rise in blood pressure is commonly seen in the early stages of stroke even in people who usually have normal blood pressure. This is a response of the body to the sudden stress of illness. However, long-standing high blood pressure is one of the common risk factors for stroke and TIA, so quite a high proportion of people with stroke and TIA have substantially elevated blood pressure readings. We'll go into more detail later about high blood pressure and how it is treated.

Blood tests

Blood is an extremely complicated fluid. In health it flows freely round the body, yet at a site of injury it will clot readily to stem any leakage. A tricky balance between the clotting and free-running nature of blood is present at any time. This balance can be disturbed for many reasons. For example, some people are born with an inherited tendency for their blood to clot too easily. More commonly some other factor is involved, such as, for example, immobility or other illness that raises the risk of clots temporarily.

Diabetes is the condition in which blood sugar (glucose) levels are raised above normal. Blood *glucose* checks are important in stroke and TIA partly because people with diabetes are at increased risk of stroke in the first place, but also because careful control of the blood glucose level is one of the factors that can improve the outcome of a person's stroke (see below).

High blood *cholesterol* is another factor that increases a person's general risk of developing hardening of the arteries and so lowering the cholesterol is an important element in the after-care of stroke (as well as in primary prevention of stroke and TIA – see chapter 10).

To cover all of the tests that possibly could be done or might be useful in assessing a person with a stroke or TIA would be a large topic and would involve more detail than is necessary here. Much depends on the total picture of a person's illness. For example, cancer of the lung can spread to the brain and the first sign might be symptoms that look exactly like a stroke. A *chest X-ray* is often done in someone who has had a stroke partly because it might show up such a diagnosis even if it were not otherwise expected.

An ECG (*electrocardiogram*) is the test in which the electrical activity of the heart is measured through wires attached to the limbs and across the chest. This can show up certain types of irregular heartbeat or may even reveal a recent heart attack, either of which can increase the tendency for clots to form within the heart, which may then break free and become lodged in the circulation of the brain.

3. Restore the blood supply (if possible)

This refers to the use of 'clot-busting drugs' that can potentially dissolve a clot within an artery. Such treatment is useful in a proportion of people who have a stroke due to artery blockage, and is explained further in the next chapter. In better-funded and equipped health care systems than the NHS, techniques are also in use that can physically remove clots from within an artery.

4. Action to minimise brain injury

The aim of good stroke care is to limit any brain damage and maximise the potential for future recovery. Experience shows that in the early stages of a stroke, particularly the first few days, attention to the following main issues may make a difference:

BLOOD PRESSURE
Although some rise in blood pressure can be caused by the stroke, excessively high blood pressure can perhaps raise the chance of further brain damage occurring. However, it may not be safe to bring down a person's blood pressure in the early stages of a stroke. Research studies are being done in this area to define what is the best approach.

OXYGEN LEVEL
An adequate flow of oxygen is essential to all living cells and, as we've seen, brain cells are particularly sensitive to oxygen lack. A stroke may adversely affect a person's breathing or lead to other problems that can lower their blood oxygen level. In turn this can increase the level of damage from the stroke. Attention to nursing care and posture (sitting up improves the ventilation of the lungs) and supplying additional oxygen when necessary by facemask helps ensure as much oxygen as possible gets through to the brain. Small oxygen-detecting probes that clip to a finger are now in

widespread use and give the nurse an instant measure of the blood oxygen level.

BLOOD SUGAR (GLUCOSE)
Diabetes is the condition in which blood glucose is abnormally high. People with diabetes have a higher risk than average of developing diseases of the heart and circulation, such as heart attack and stroke, so someone with diabetes is more likely than average to suffer a stroke. It is also common for diabetes to be diagnosed for the first time when someone has a stroke. Possibly the acute stress on the body caused by having a stroke can make a person who is not diabetic develop high blood glucose for the first time. Although brain cells are completely dependent on glucose for their energy, very high glucose levels appear to be damaging to brain cells. People who have had a stroke and whose blood glucose level goes up and stays up appear to do less well than those whose blood glucose levels are controlled more tightly. To achieve this control it is sometimes necessary to give insulin by injections or a drip for a while.

BODY TEMPERATURE CONTROL
The presence of a fever is associated with an increase in the amount of brain tissue that is affected by a particular stroke. Fever is most commonly due to infection, and someone with a stroke may be at increased risk of developing, for example, an infection in the chest if their overall condition is poor or their swallowing reflex has been impaired, increasing their chance of something 'going down the wrong way'. The first attention a fever needs is therefore to diagnose its cause and treat it, with antibiotics if necessary. However, a fever in stroke may also reflect a direct effect of the stroke on the body's 'thermostat', which consists of specialised brain cells deep in the centre of the brain. Drugs such as paracetamol act to lower body temperature, hence their widespread use in general fever control. Keeping

down a fever may help limit the extent of a stroke.

Lowering of the body's temperature reduces its need for oxygen and energy, which is why there are occasional remarkable stories of people recovering from prolonged immersion in icy water. It is not yet known whether deliberate reduction of the body temperature by more sophisticated means could be used as a type of stroke treatment, but this is one line of current research.

SWALLOWING, NUTRITION AND FLUID REPLACEMENT
Although we do not ordinarily give it any thought, swallowing is a complicated process involving many muscles of the face and throat, all acting in a co-ordinated way. Strokes affecting the circulation to the back of the brain (the brain stem) may impair a person's ability to swallow properly, which can lead to several important problems. First is the risk of inhaling food or fluids into the lung, with the consequent risk of lung infection. Secondly, poor swallowing will lead to reduced oral intake of food and fluids, which in turn can cause dehydration and inadequate nutrition. All of these are detrimental to the person's health and can lead to serious consequences.

Particularly in the first week after a stroke nursing staff should regularly assess a person's ability to swallow. This can be done by carefully observing how the person copes with small sips of water, while checking that the swallowing muscles in the throat are active. If there is any uncertainty then the speech and language therapist is usually the person who has particular expertise in swallow assessment. When swallowing problems are present a number of extra steps may be needed, from basic help with feeding through to giving extra fluids via a drip into the veins or even to the use of a feeding tube passed into the stomach. Nutritional advice from the dietician is likely to be required if normal food cannot be managed. Poor nutrition and dehydration can increase the size and impact of a stroke, whereas detecting and managing this aspect of care early on ensures that people with stroke do not suffer avoidable worsening of their condition. Further information on longer-term assistance with feeding in people who have suffered a stroke is in chapter 9.

BRAIN-PROTECTING DRUGS

Laboratory work suggests that it may be possible to use drugs to increase the resistance of brain cells to the sorts of 'injury' caused by stroke. No such medicines have ever reached the stage of being suitable for clinical use, but it is an area of active research.

5. Good general care

INFORMATION

A stroke is a frightening event for anyone, including the family. Strokes can also impair a person's ability to communicate, although not necessarily to understand or to be bewildered or anxious. In the initial stages of the illness there is usually a great deal of uncertainty about what will happen next, and even more about what will happen in the long run. Nursing and medical staff can help a lot by doing their best to explain what they know about the person's condition, about what the test results mean and what the treatments are that are being used. Not everyone wants to know everything all the time, but most people want to know more than they are routinely told, and they are better off for having that information.

Information is a vital component of the support needed by people with stroke, their carers, friends and families, and it should not be one-way. People who have had a stroke, and the relevant people around them, need and benefit from the opportunity to air their own views about progress, problems and care decisions.

EARLY MOBILISATION

Bed can be a dangerous place to be in for too long. Early mobilisation helps reduce the chances of developing chest infections, blood clots in the legs (deep vein thrombosis), skin pressure problems, constipation, muscle weakness, joint stiffness and diminished morale. Just how quickly after a stroke someone can start to mobilise obviously depends on their individual circumstances, but day one need not be too soon.

EARLY REHABILITATION
For the same reasons, rehabilitation should be planned and acted upon as soon as this is feasible. Within stroke care teams, the various professions will be organised to become involved. Multidisciplinary teams that communicate regularly, with each other and with patients and their carers, achieve better results.

Difficult decisions

As with all medical conditions, hard choices sometimes have to be made. Although, as was mentioned early on, some people with major stroke damage make surprisingly good recoveries, this is uncommon. It may become clear in the early phase of someone's stroke that although he or she has survived the initial event, the extent of the brain injury is severe. Predicting how much recovery someone is likely to make from such a position can be almost impossible. It can be a little easier to confirm that the level of brain damage is such that substantial recovery is unlikely.

Modern medical technology can keep severely brain-injured people alive for very considerable lengths of time. Inevitably we will see increasing numbers, as time goes on, of individuals who have had a stroke and whose quality of life is questionable and for whom decisions such as the appropriateness of resuscitation will vex their loved ones and carers alike. So individual is this matter that one can do little more than air it and confirm its importance.

Decisions on how hard to try and maintain someone's life against a background of a severe stroke are hard for everyone to make. Often it is after a stroke or other similarly incapacitating illness that this important topic is discussed for the first time. This is usually the most difficult time to talk about it – everyone is in shock at the change in circumstances and the person with the stroke is least likely to be able to take part in the discussion.

Increasingly, however, people are planning ahead and putting down their thoughts about how they wish to be treated should an illness like a stroke prevent them from expressing their wishes.

Early stroke care facilities in the UK

There are many different aspects to good stroke care, and when they are all addressed well this leads to better outcomes. Specifically trained nurses, doctors and other health professionals working within a dedicated stroke unit are more able to cover all these issues than staff who have to divide their attention among people with a wide range of medical problems, as is the usual case on a busy medical ward.

As was referred to earlier in this chapter, the provision of services for the rapid assessment of people who have had a TIA or stroke is still patchy and short of ideal across the UK. Some areas have good services that respond well and quickly, while others have poor services with unacceptably slow response times. In November 2005 the National Audit Office published the results of its assessment of stroke services in England. Similar reviews are taking place across the other regions of the UK. These reviews reveal deficiencies and call for improvement. When such calls circulate only within the health professions then a certain amount does tend to happen, eventually. When a well-informed public gets to know that they may be receiving a second-class service this tends to result in a call for the allocation of resources more speedily.

Key Points

- In the early management of stroke rapid medical assessment is essential. This usually means hospital admission.
- TIA may also need hospital admission but rapid-access outpatient clinics can suffice if well organised.
- The role of initial tests is to establish as precisely as possible the type of stroke and possible contributing factors.
- CT or MRI brain scanning should be done within 48 hours of the onset of symptoms to distinguish strokes due to artery blockage (ischaemic) from those due to bleeding (haemorrhagic).
- A sound wave device (ultrasound, Duplex Doppler) is the commonest method of scanning the carotid arteries as well as the heart for possible sources of clots that give rise to ischaemic stroke.
- The outcome for a person following a stroke is improved if certain factors such as blood pressure, blood glucose, oxygen levels and body temperature are kept under control.
- Early attention to fluid and food intake, and watching out for swallowing difficulties, are also very important.
- Everyone needs good quality information and feedback about what is going on.

Chapter 7

Treatment for stroke due to artery blockage (ischaemic stroke)

The previous chapter has outlined that one of the most important tasks in the early stages following the onset of symptoms of a stroke is to be sure what type of stroke it is, i.e. whether it is due to blockage of, or bleeding from, a brain artery. Eighty-five per cent of strokes are due to blockage of a brain artery. The medical term for all of them is 'ischaemic strokes'. An ischaemic stroke can be caused by a blood clot that forms inside the artery of the brain (thrombotic stroke), or by a clot that forms somewhere else in the body and travels to the brain (embolic stroke).

Recapping information from chapter 2, an artery may become blocked in one of two ways:

1. **Internal build-up**: As we get older the lining of our arteries gets thicker or 'furred up', so the width of the available channel

for blood gets narrower. Eventually the artery can close up altogether. This is what is meant by 'hardening of the arteries'. This is the most common of all types of stroke.
2. *Jamming*: A piece of material, such as a blood clot, travels from another part of the circulation and gets jammed in a brain artery, stopping blood from getting through. Usually the source of the clot is the heart or an area within the main (carotid) arteries in the neck.

Aspirin

As far as strokes are concerned the property that makes aspirin useful is its effect on the tiny particles within blood called platelets. These minute cells, the smallest in the blood, have a number of roles in stopping bleeding from blood vessels. Platelets are present in high numbers in the blood and normally they circulate freely. When the blood clotting process is triggered, such as at the site of a cut, platelets become 'sticky' and clump together. Such masses of platelets are an important component of blood clots.

Aspirin has the remarkable property of stopping platelets becoming sticky. It thereby reduces the tendency of blood to clot. This action is called its 'anti-platelet effect'. A small number of other drugs also have an anti-platelet effect and are used in stroke treatment, but aspirin was the first in this family tree and remains the most common. It offers a small degree of protection against further stroke (about 18–22 per cent less chance of stroke developing over two years).

In stopping platelets from clumping together aspirin reduces the ability of blood to form clots. Aspirin can therefore make a cut bleed for longer. In the case of a bleeding artery in the brain aspirin might tend to worsen the degree of bleeding. It therefore becomes obvious why it is important to distinguish between the two main types of stroke. In the case of ischaemic stroke aspirin has a beneficial effect, reducing the tendency of more clot to form within a brain artery. In the case of haemorrhagic stroke aspirin might make the situation worse. Only a brain scan can really tell the difference. (However, recent research evidence suggests that the possible adverse effect of using aspirin in haemorrhagic stroke is actually very small.)

> Aspirin, started within 48 hours of the onset of an ischaemic stroke, slightly reduces the impact of the stroke. Unless someone is allergic to aspirin or has previously had a bad reaction to it then everyone with an ischaemic stroke should be started on aspirin as soon as the diagnosis is clear, and certainly within 48 hours.

Aspirin is a long-acting drug and needs to be taken only once daily. A standard aspirin tablet contains 300mg (milligrams) of aspirin and one tablet daily is usually used for the first dose. The anti-platelet effect of aspirin is also present at a lower dose, and lower doses are less likely to give side effects. It is therefore usual practice to then change to low dose aspirin (75mg daily) after the first dose. Aspirin given in this way helps a little to protect against another stroke happening.

The main potential side effect from aspirin is irritation of the lining of the stomach. This can cause indigestion, or an ulcer or even bleeding from the stomach. To minimise the chances of such side effects, apart from using low dose aspirin, it can also help to use anti-ulcer medicines at the same time, which help to protect the stomach.

Other anti-platelet drugs

Two other anti-platelet drugs are commonly used in stroke treatment:

DIPYRIDAMOLE MODIFIED RELEASE

This may be given in addition to aspirin and some current expert guidelines recommend doing so for two years following a stroke. The brand name of dipyridamole modified release is Persantin® Retard.

CLOPIDOGREL

An alternative to aspirin. It can also cause side effects on the stomach. The brand name of clopidogrel is Plavix®.

Research continues into combinations of anti-platelet drugs to see which gives the best results with minimum side effects. The important point is that their use should be seriously considered in everyone who has had a stroke or TIA, and the vast majority of those people should take such medicine regularly.

'Clot-dissolving' drugs

One of the most important advances in new medicines over the past several years has been the development of 'clot-dissolving' or 'clot-busting' drugs. The medical term for these drugs is 'thrombolytics' (from *thrombus*, meaning clot and *lysis*, meaning dissolve). These drugs boost the power of the blood's own clot-dissolving ability and given quickly enough they can even clear a newly blocked artery. Thrombolytic drugs have found an important place in the early treatment of heart attacks, as by far the commonest cause of heart attacks is blockage of one of the arteries supplying blood back to the heart muscle. This is therefore very similar to what happens in the brain in ischaemic stroke.

Like aspirin, a thrombolytic drug will worsen bleeding in the case of a haemorrhagic stroke. In fact, thrombolytic drugs have a more powerful effect than aspirin in this respect, so one needs to be very sure that a stroke is not due to bleeding before using a clot-dissolving medicine. Such worries have not been an issue in their use in heart attacks as bleeding into the heart muscle is a problem that very rarely arises.

ALTEPLASE
There are several clot-dissolving drugs available. Alteplase is the one for which the most research evidence is presently available when used in stroke. When given within three hours of the onset of stroke symptoms (the earlier the better) to carefully selected people (i.e. avoiding people who may react badly to a thrombolytic drug for other reasons), alteplase improves the outcome of stroke. Specifically it reduces the extent of disability suffered by stroke survivors.

Alteplase administration does not increase the total number of people who survive a stroke, because about 5 per cent of people who are given the drug suffer increased bleeding to a degree that proves fatal. This increase in mortality balances out the benefits in survival experienced by other people given alteplase. Alteplase is given only by injection. Its brand name is Actilyse®.

One can see from this that the use of these powerful medicines is not without risks and difficulties. More research continues to try and clarify how we can use thrombolytic drugs to the best advantage.

One can also see clearly that clot-dissolving drugs can only be used when there are well-organised medical services capable of admitting patients to hospital very soon after the onset of their stroke, scanning them almost immediately and then carefully selecting those people who, on the basis of current knowledge, are likely to benefit from the treatment. This implies exceptionally well-organised local stroke services and, as we've mentioned more than once, that does not yet exist in a consistent way across the UK. In fact, the restrictions on the use of alteplase go further at present because its use across the UK is part of an international research effort, so the number of centres able to offer the treatment is very limited.

It seems very likely, however, that as knowledge about thrombolytic drugs increases and services improve we will see an expansion of the use of this treatment for stroke over the coming years.

Treatment to 'thin the blood'

There is another major form of treatment available that reduces the tendency of blood to clot. Drugs that do this are called 'anticoagulants'. There are two main forms of anticoagulant drug in current use.

HEPARIN
This works right away but must be given by injection.

WARFARIN
This works when given by mouth in tablet form but takes several days to build up its effect.

These drugs are popularly thought of as 'thinning the blood'. In fact they do not do so – people who don't take heparin or warfarin have blood that is just as runny as those who do! However, the effect of anticoagulant drugs is to slow down the time it takes for clots to form in the blood when the 'clotting process' would normally go into action, for example at the site of a cut.

Unlike aspirin, which works by reducing the tendency of platelets to stick together, heparin and warfarin work by slowing the complicated series of chemical reactions that go on when blood clots.

Anticoagulant drugs tend not to be used in the early treatment of ischaemic stroke. The reason is that although they reduce the chance of more clots occurring they also increase the chance that an ischaemic stroke will change into one in which there is bleeding (i.e. it becomes a haemorrhagic stroke). The disadvantages outweigh the advantages. An exception is when someone has an irregular heartbeat of the type called atrial fibrillation (this is explained further in chapter 10). Here the risk of small clots forming in the blood is much increased and the early and continued use of anticoagulants is beneficial.

Carotid artery surgery

One important source of blood clots that cause strokes is furring up of one or both carotid arteries in the neck. The material that builds up in arteries in this way is fragile and can break off, sending fragments into the blood that can get stuck 'downstream' – in the brain.

The typical place for such blockage to build up is the point around the angle of the jaw where the main carotid artery, sending blood up the neck, divides into two. The deeper branch thus formed is the internal carotid artery, which goes to the Circle of Willis to supply the brain (chapter 4). The other branch (external carotid artery) supplies blood to the face. Twenty to thirty per cent of people who have a TIA or ischaemic stroke have narrowing of the carotid artery in this region. Investigation of the carotid arteries is first done with ultrasound (chapter 6). If this indicates significant blockage more sophisticated tests can be done that allow accurate measurement of the degree of narrowing of the artery, but some surgical units will operate on the ultrasound findings alone.

People who have had a stroke or TIA and who have 70–99 per cent or more narrowing of the carotid artery (i.e. the available channel for blood is 1–30 per cent of normal) benefit from surgery to remove the thickened lining. (Surgery is only useful to the patient if the artery still has some blood flowing through it. Completely closed arteries are left alone.) Although easier said than done, the technique is that the surgeon isolates the 'furred up' section of the carotid artery with clamps and then opens it up along its length over the narrowed segment. The internal lining can be carefully dissected away, the debris washed out and the much cleaner and wider artery sewn back up again before the clamps are removed and an improved flow of blood is let through. The technique is called 'carotid endarterectomy'. A 'rebore' is a less technical term but gives an idea of what is done.

Carotid endarterectomy has negligible benefits for narrowing that is less severe, down to about 50 per cent. If the degree of carotid artery narrowing is less than 50 per cent (i.e. the available channel for blood is 50 per cent or more that of normal) then endarterectomy is not beneficial. Carotid surgery is a major procedure. People have to be fit enough to have it done, which includes having recovered from their stroke. There are accompanying risks, including a 3–5 per cent chance of another stroke occurring at or soon after the operation.

The timing of carotid endarterectomy is important and the best results are obtained when it is done within a short time of the stroke, preferably well within a month – a target that is yet to be achieved in most areas of the NHS. As with clot-dissolving treatment, stroke services must be well organised and able to respond quickly if people with stroke are to get what we currently understand to be the best treatment.

Key Points

- Strokes due to blockage of a brain artery (ischaemic stroke) are the commonest type.
- Medicines that stop blood platelets from sticking together are useful in the early stages of ischaemic stroke and whenever possible they should be started within 48 hours.
- Aspirin is the commonest anti-platelet drug. Others include dipyridamole modified release and clopidogrel.

- Medicines to help dissolve blood clots, called thrombolytic drugs, are useful in a selected group of people who have an ischaemic stroke.
- Thrombolytic drugs can reduce eventual disability from stroke but do not reduce the overall likelihood of dying from a severe stroke.
- Alteplase is the thrombolytic drug currently licensed for such use.
- Drugs that reduce the general tendency of blood to clot (anticoagulants), namely heparin and warfarin, are not useful in the early stages of treatment of ischaemic stroke.
- In the case of a stroke due to hardening of the carotid artery, early surgery to clear the blockage may be beneficial if the artery is more than 50 per cent blocked, and particularly if it is more than 70 per cent blocked.

Chapter 8

Treatment for stroke due to artery bleeding (haemorrhagic stroke)

Background information

Haemorrhage into the brain carries with it a high risk of damage to brain tissue. People who have a haemorrhagic stroke are four to five times less common than those with thrombotic stroke, but they have a higher risk of dying – up to 50 per cent do so within the first month. People with haemorrhagic stroke tend to be less well as a group and home management is not usually an option for them unless only palliative treatment is the aim, i.e. they are already too unwell for active treatment to be appropriate.

Conversely, people who survive a haemorrhagic stroke tend to have less long-term disability than those who survive an ischaemic stroke.

In the majority (about 75 per cent) of haemorrhagic strokes the bleeding occurs into the brain. In 25 per cent the bleeding is into the fluid-filled space around the brain (subarachnoid haemorrhage).

The main risk factor for haemorrhagic stroke is, as with ischaemic stroke, having high blood pressure. Other risks include the taking of anticoagulants (including when this is to reduce the risk of ischaemic stroke: there are pros and cons to most medical decisions). In subarachnoid haemorrhage there is an increased chance that the bleed has arisen from a berry aneurysm (chapter 2).

Drugs of abuse such as cocaine, ecstasy and amphetamines are responsible for a small number of haemorrhagic and ischaemic strokes each year in younger people. Cocaine irritates the lining of arteries, making rupture of the artery possible. Ecstasy and amphetamines can cause sudden, very high increases in the user's blood pressure, which may open a weak point in one of the arteries of the brain.

Aims of treatment

In ischaemic stroke the treatment is aimed at stopping further blood clotting, and even at dissolving any clots that have already formed. In haemorrhagic stroke one wants to do the opposite and encourage clotting, at least at the point of leakage from the ruptured blood vessel. The basic principles of first aid also say that to stop bleeding you need to block off the bleeding source, by applying pressure or a tourniquet for example. Put simply, these are indeed the two main approaches to haemorrhagic stroke treatment. However, in practice it isn't that simple.

ENCOURAGING BLOOD TO CLOT
Treatment to encourage blood to clot does exist but its role in the treatment of haemorrhagic stroke is still very much at the research

stage. A recent study has shown promising results for the use of a clot-promoting drug given within three hours of the onset of the haemorrhage. Such treatments are only likely to limit the area of damage rather than promote healing of a damaged area and much more work is needed before we can be sure of the value of this type of treatment.

DIRECT APPROACH TO THE BLEEDING ARTERY
Desirable as it may seem to clip off a bleeding artery in some way, when the bleeding is deep within the skull the task of getting to the bleeding source without at the same time causing damage to healthy brain is extremely difficult. In practical terms, therefore, it is not usually possible for a specialist surgeon (neurosurgeon) to help the majority of people with a brain haemorrhage in such a direct way.

Subarachnoid haemorrhage is, to some extent, an exception. You may remember from chapter 2 that in a subarachnoid haemorrhage bleeding occurs into the fluid that bathes the brain and spinal cord and that this condition is particularly associated with a 'berry aneurysm'. Investigation of the blood flow through the brain at the time of the haemorrhage may reveal such an aneurysm, and sometimes these are accessible for the neurosurgeon to reach. Other techniques are now used in which specially designed metal (platinum) coils are threaded along the artery and into the aneurysm. There the coil blocks the flow of blood into the aneurysm, which seals it off. This 'minimally invasive' procedure is done under X-ray screening and avoids skull-opening surgery.

Other surgical aspects of brain haemorrhage

Unless there is an escape route for leaking blood it collects around the point of bleeding. That is basically what a bruise is – blood in the tissues. When a lot of blood collects at a point it congeals into a jelly-like mass called a haematoma (*hee-ma-toh-ma*). A haematoma within the skull is, of course, most unwelcome, as the skull cannot expand. Healthy brain tissue therefore becomes squeezed by the haematoma.

It is possible for a neurosurgeon to operate and drain a haematoma within the brain but the results of a recent large research study showed that this was generally not a useful action to take. There were some exceptions, notably when the haematoma was in the region around the cerebellum (chapter 3). As the brain stem is also in this region, compression from a haematoma could potentially cause major problems, such as stopping the person breathing. A neurosurgeon's opinion would therefore be called for if someone had a stroke and had a haematoma in such a position. The decision to operate would still be a difficult one, with much attached risk.

Other than these specific circumstances, therefore, surgical treatment is generally not of great value in haemorrhagic stroke.

General aspects of treatment

These were outlined in chapter 6 and apply to all types of stroke.

BLOOD PRESSURE

Avoidance of very high blood pressure is probably also of value in haemorrhagic stroke. Again though, the balance needs to be struck between lowering the blood pressure to a safe level and not lowering it so much that an adequate blood flow fails to get through to the rest of the brain.

BLOOD GLUCOSE

High blood glucose levels may increase the size of a haematoma, reinforcing the need to keep the blood glucose well controlled.

PREVENTION OF FITS

Stroke of either type is associated with an increased risk of fits, particularly within the first 24 hours. People with many fits from a stroke may do less well, and giving drugs to prevent fits (anticonvulsants) is therefore potentially helpful. They may only be needed for a few weeks.

Key Points

- Haemorrhagic stroke is less common than ischaemic stroke but is more likely to be fatal.
- There are fewer options for treatment than in ischaemic stroke at the present time.
- General supportive care is the most important aspect of treatment.
- Medical treatment to limit the extent of the bleeding is one area of research.
- Surgery is generally not helpful except in certain situations, such as subarachnoid bleeding or bleeding around the cerebellum. The opinion of a neurosurgeon is needed in those circumstances.

Chapter 9

Rehabilitation

The majority of people affected by stroke will be taken by surprise by it. In all probability they will have spent little or no time thinking about stroke before it happens to them. Quite probably they will not have a great deal of knowledge about what the consequences of having a stroke are likely to be. If they do have an image of the aftermath of a stroke it will almost certainly be negative. Common views are that strokes are always very disabling, that working after a stroke would be out of the question and that if you have one stroke you are bound to have another one.

In fact, although the impact of stroke can be enormous, a high proportion of people make a good recovery. Many of working age do get back to employment. Most people have only one stroke – such is the value of 'secondary prevention'.

Many people, none the less, do remain disabled to a greater or lesser extent and some adaptation to life after a stroke is always necessary. Maximising one's recovery, adapting to problems and learning to live with what can't be improved is the process of rehabilitation. It's a journey of the body and of the mind. It can, and usually does, involve not only the person who has had the stroke but their family, friends and colleagues.

Rehabilitation is, or ought to be, 'patient-centred'. The most important person in the rehabilitation team is the person who has had the stroke, and the help he or she needs is an individual matter. In the rest of this chapter some coverage is given to each of the main issues that can arise after a stroke. Mention is also made of the various members of the rehabilitation team who are involved, or can be, in helping someone recover from a stroke.

Main areas of potential need in rehabilitation

A complete list of every possible area of impact that could be relevant to stroke would be very lengthy. The following is a selection of the most important:

1. Mobility and movement
2. Communication and speech
3. Intellectual impairment
4. Body awareness
5. Nutrition and swallowing
6. Emotions and relationships
7. Continence
8. Work
9. Driving
10. Reducing the risk of further stroke (this major topic has the next chapter to itself)

1. MOBILITY AND MOVEMENT
As we've seen, damage to the nerves that control muscle

movement is one of the main possible effects of a stroke. This might range from a localised muscle weakness that is so small as not to be troublesome, all the way to the complete loss of power down one side of the body.

Combinations of problems
The impact of loss of function in the arms is greater if it involves the dominant arm. For most people that means their right arm. Right-sided power loss implies left-sided brain damage, and potentially such a stroke may therefore also involve the nearby Broca's speech area. One can see, therefore, that combinations of disabilities are not uncommon after a stroke. Some combinations are potentially more disabling than others.

Balance
Although it is what we do naturally as human beings, standing and walking about on two feet is neither easy nor very safe. That can clearly be seen in the efforts of a child learning to walk. It's equally obvious that the would-be toddler is not put off by any number of falls in his or her determination to master the activity. Walking requires strong muscles that are able to move quickly as well as a highly efficient balance control centre. Mobility is vulnerable in stroke for various possible reasons. The loss of power in a leg is the most obvious one, but damage to the cerebellum or brain stem may disable our ability to balance or control our other muscles with sufficient precision to allow us to keep on an even keel.

Muscle weakness
The initial effect of stroke on a muscle is to weaken it. This occurs because the normal nerve commands to the muscle that would tell it to contract do not get through. Without use muscles quickly lose their bulk and become weaker. In the longer term affected muscles may contract or go into spasm. In the case of those muscles that have the job of moving a particular joint this can result in stiffness

and a reduction in the range of movement of the joint as well as weakness.

Physiotherapy
The **physiotherapist** is the key health worker for matters relating to muscle activity and control. Programmes of exercise designed to regain as much activity as possible, as well as to prevent the tightening up of joints, can often be started very early in stroke – even on the first day. Work started by the hospital physiotherapy service while an in-patient is then continued by the community-based physiotherapists. Most of the time they will work from a centre to which the patient travels for their sessions. For a small proportion of people for whom travelling is impractical they can provide physiotherapy input at home.

An important part of the success of physiotherapy, in fact the key element, is the degree to which the person receiving the physiotherapy engages with it. Physiotherapy is not something you 'have done to you'. It is much more of a two-way effort, in which the therapist teaches the sorts of things that you can do to help yourself. Often that will still require the help of others, whether physiotherapist or family member, to be successful. This will be particularly so in the early stages when recovery may seem to be slow. In the case of preventing muscles from 'seizing up' and joints from tightening someone who has little movement at a joint will require help from someone else to put the joint regularly through a full range of movement. (This is called passive exercise as someone else is supplying the muscle power.)

Common areas of difficulty in the early stages after a stroke, and those on which the physiotherapists will concentrate their efforts, are dressing, feeding, walking, bathing and toileting. Stair-climbing ability is important for most people even if they live in stairless houses and may be a particular challenge for some people after a stroke.

Coping at home

Unless someone is lucky enough to quickly regain full mobility and balance after their stroke it is likely that when they get home a number of problems that didn't exist beforehand will crop up. The loose rug in the living room may become a major trip hazard for someone whose stroke has left her with a tendency for a foot to drag. The bathroom taps may suddenly become impossible to budge with a weaker hand. The toilet seat might be too low to get up from without assistance, the front doorsteps a barrier to getting in and out of the house – and so on. Nursing staff and physiotherapists have quite a lot to do with picking up such problem areas but the **occupational therapist (OT)** normally takes the lead role. 'Occupational' in this sense is not about work but about how people function in relation to their environment – in particular their home.

The OT in hospital will co-operate with the physiotherapist in assessing how someone copes with the various activities of daily living. When home discharge is on the cards they or the community OT will accompany the person who has had the stroke on a visit to their home to see what sort of assistance might be required. This could range from minor adjustments to the layout of the furniture, through the strategic placement of handrails to the need for door ramps or even major adaptation of the house to make it suitable. Funding assistance for some of these works may be available from the local authority and advice on this is usually sought through a **social worker**. It is common for a social worker to see a person who might need such help while they are still in hospital and then liaise with the local social work office, but they can also be asked to help at some later stage if the need does not become apparent until the person is home.

Persistence pays off

Stroke recovery can be very slow and prolonged. It's worth remembering this when months, or even years, have gone by and problems still remain. The limits of any person's ability to recover are not set out in any book of rules. No matter how severe the effects of a stroke no doctor, physiotherapist or anyone else can say with confidence that a particular ability is lost forever. By means that we are still far from understanding, the brain is capable of findings ways to cope. This is worth recalling when the effort of trying to recover appears to show little return.

2. COMMUNICATION AND SPEECH

We saw earlier how the left side of the brain tends to be dominant in processing the information from the senses and in handling language and speech. Speech and language are enormously important to us and a substantial amount of our 'brainpower' is given over to handling these functions. They are, however, only part of what we use to communicate with each other. Non-verbal communication – 'body language' – makes up a substantial proportion of the total.

Difficulties in language understanding – 'aphasia'

Especially in left-hemisphere strokes there may be difficulties at any stage in receiving, making sense of and giving out messages, whether by speech or any other method. Right-hemisphere strokes can also give rise to communication difficulty, in which case the non-verbal element may be more affected than the speech side.

'Aphasia' (*ay-faze-ee-ah*) is the medical term for this general problem. Over a third of people with stroke suffer some degree of aphasia initially.

It can help a little in understanding aphasia to break it into two main types:

- ***Expressive aphasia*** is the commonest. In this type the person who has had the stroke understands what is said to him perfectly well. His difficulty is in bringing together the words that allow him to express what he wants to say back.

In expressive aphasia speech is therefore hesitant and often does not make sense. It can be accompanied by much frustration both on the part of the person who has had the stroke and the listener trying to understand him. Such frustrations are easily made worse if the listener assumes, as too often happens, a patronising attitude that makes it fairly obvious he thinks the speaker is a bit deaf or stupid.
- ***Receptive aphasia*** is less common. Here the person does not understand what is being said to him. He is able to speak fluently back but the content of his speech may not make much sense.

Difficulties in speaking – dysarthria

A stroke may affect the muscles of the tongue and voice-box (larynx) and the muscles of breathing, as well as the co-ordination of all of them, and these need to work properly together to produce speech. Speech impairment due to problems with the 'machinery' of speaking is called 'dysarthria' (*dis-arth-ree-ah*). Although dysarthria and aphasia may occur together they need not do so. Someone who only has dysarthria understands language perfectly and knows exactly what he wants to say back. His difficulty is in producing the right sounds. As an illustration of the difference, someone who is trying to speak with a mouthful of food has temporary dysarthria.

Speech and language therapy

The **speech and language therapist (SLT)** is the expert in diagnosing and treating problems in this area. The SLT can differentiate and treat speech problems due to understanding (aphasia) and those due to the mechanics of speech (dysarthria). Often there is some element of both.

The presence of aphasia and/or dysarthria has major influences on how disabling a particular stroke can be. Their presence can considerably reduce a person's quality of life and adversely affect their relationships and their employability even if they have no other disability from their stroke. Depression is much more common in people who have speech and language problems after a stroke.

The degree to which aphasia and dysarthria can be overcome is very variable. Increasingly it is possible for the speech and language therapist to call upon technological aids to help someone express themselves properly, such as, for example, speech generating devices where dysarthria is the major issue. Through making an accurate personal assessment of a person's needs the SLT may see ways of getting round some aspects of their disability. For example, someone might be better able to understand pictures than word-based information, in which case drawings and simple diagrams may achieve more than written information.

As you might expect, the benefits achievable using speech and language therapy are related in part to the amount of time devoted to the treatment. To gain the best results in people who have severe aphasia requires several hours of input each week, extending over many months. It can be difficult to achieve such a level of input as, like most such health professionals, there is a shortage of trained speech and language therapists in the UK. Additional help from family and from voluntary stroke services can be very useful supplements to the input of the SLT.

3. INTELLECTUAL IMPAIRMENT

Language gets special attention because of its importance but impairment of other aspects of a person's intellectual abilities can of course occur as a result of a stroke. For example, there may be issues with memory loss, impaired judgement and decision-making, poor attention span and reduced problem-solving abilities.

GPs and other health workers can use simple screening tools, such as questionnaires, to help detect when people have significant intellectual impairment. However, these are relatively crude and can miss important details. Ideally people need help from **psychologists** trained in stroke rehabilitation to help diagnose the difficulties and provide strategies for dealing with them. Such services are not very widely available as there is a considerable shortage of suitably qualified psychologists in the UK.

Just how much recovery is likely to occur in someone left with severe intellectual impairment after a stroke is almost impossible to predict. As with other aspects of stroke treatment one should not give up trying and time can eventually reap rewards. Even if the extent of the improvement is slight, skilled psychology input can help the carers to cope, and this is worth a lot.

4. BODY AWARENESS

Stroke involving the sides of the brain (parietal lobes) in particular can cause significant problems with a person's ability to recognise their own body. The example given in chapter 3 was of someone failing to recognise that his arm, paralysed from a stroke, is part of his own body. Such 'neglect' of a part of the body can give rise to various difficulties such as injury of the neglected part. That risk may be increased if the stroke has altered the person's ability to feel pain.

Neglect of visual information may increase the risk of injury in other ways. For example, a car approaching on the 'neglected side' might not be perceived as a risk when crossing the road. It may alternatively be that the car is not seen if a stroke has involved an area of the occipital lobe, at the back of the brain, where information from the eyes is received and processed. A pattern of stroke that can result is the loss of one half of the visual field of each eye, the blind side being the same in each eye.

Little can be done to improve such lost function, unfortunately. It helps to know that the problem exists, and for others to remember it. Thus one might know to approach someone from his or her 'good side' or to shake hands with the non-neglected one. Special precautions may be necessary to avoid injury in hazardous environments such as around the cooker, and to ensure that hot water is not allowed to get too hot to scald before it is noticed, etc. This is another area where the occupational therapist is best placed to advise.

5. NUTRITION AND SWALLOWING

Normal swallowing is a complicated business. A great many muscles of the face, tongue and throat are involved in chewing food properly, bringing it to the back of the throat, and then swallowing it, while at the same time muscles close the top of the airway tube, above the voice-box (larynx) to ensure that we don't inhale food as it goes down. After a stroke there can be problems with any part of this process. The main danger that results is that food may get into the airways. This greatly increases the risk of a potentially serious chest infection. If someone cannot swallow properly they will also quickly become dehydrated and malnourished.

Assessment of swallowing is therefore an important early part of the care a person receives when they have had a stroke. Initially this is likely to be done on the ward by the nurse, but the speech and language therapist is the expert and will advise if there is any uncertainty. The nurse gives a small amount of water to drink while the person sits up. Signs of problems would include the absence of any swallowing action, a cough during swallowing, gurgling noises or shortness of breath.

Treatment of swallowing difficulty may need the input of nursing and medical staff and the dietician as well as the speech and language therapist. Strategies need to be adapted to the circumstances. For some people careful attention to the position of their head and the size of the mouthfuls may be enough to let them eat a normal diet. Others may require their food to be rendered more easily swallowed by pureeing it. Fluids can be made a little less runny by adding thickeners, which allows more control over swallowing them.

Feeding tubes

If, despite such measures, problems still remain then it may be necessary to use some form of assisted feeding. This can be done by passing a thin tube into the stomach, either through the nose and all the way down the gullet (naso-gastric tube) or by placing a feeding tube directly through the skin and into the stomach. The latter can be done under local anaesthetic and is easier to do than it may sound. The proper name for this direct feeding tube is 'Percutaneous Endoscopic Gastrotomy', better known to all as a 'PEG' tube. Through either the nasal tube or the PEG tube adequate amounts of nutritionally complete liquid feeds can be given easily.

The advantage of the PEG tube is that it is out of the way when not in use. Fine feeding tubes that go through the nose work well enough but they need to be strapped to the face and are visible all the time. They can be irritating and are prone to getting in the way when the person is being washed. If, additionally, the stroke has impaired someone's ability to understand what the purpose of the tube is then they might just haul it up. That might also, in the case of someone who cannot communicate easily, be a signal that they don't want such intervention.

Recent research has indicated that people given PEG tube feeding have poorer outcomes compared to those given naso-gastric feeding. The reasons for the differences are not entirely clear. It could be that people who receive PEG tube feeding are as a group more dependent, more likely to be cared for in institutions and have a poorer quality of life in general. PEG tubes are useful and can make long-term assisted feeding more manageable, but naso-gastric tube feeding is the preferred option when someone needs help with their nutrition in the early stages after their stroke.

Ethical issues

As interventions of this nature tend to be necessary in people with more severe strokes ethical dilemmas can arise in their use. Of course, one should try to gain the views of the person who has had the stroke about whether they wish to have such treatment. But that is not always easily done, and may be impossible if the person is very ill and unable to communicate. In such circumstances the views of the family are very important, but medical staff may still have to act as arbiters in decisions on how much intervention is reasonable.

6. EMOTIONS AND RELATIONSHIPS

Depression

Emotional disturbances, particularly depression, are common after stroke. They are more likely when progress following the stroke has been slow, when the length of time in hospital has been long (which usually means that the level of disability following the stroke is high) and when there are communication difficulties such as expressive aphasia.

Mood changes

Stroke can also cause someone's mood to apparently be highly changeable. For example, someone might burst into tears for no good reason (alternatively they might start laughing inappropriately). This 'emotional lability' can therefore give misleading signals – it may be that in neither case is the person actually unhappy or happy. The effect of the stroke has been to disconnect the usual signs of emotion that we are used to seeing, from what is actually happening to the person's mood. At first it can be disconcerting to have to re-interpret someone's emotional reactions, so powerful is our own natural response to such things. Understanding that emotional lability can happen after stroke and learning how to deal with it takes time and effort.

The diagnosis of depression and other mood disturbance can therefore be more difficult following a stroke. Knowing that it is common, however, means that it must be looked for. Antidepressant medication is effective when given to people who definitely have depression following stroke. Other types of treatment, such as psychological counselling and other non-drug types of treatment, have been less well studied in stroke but are probably not very effective on their own.

Emotional difficulties are not necessarily confined to the person who has had the stroke. Their partner and family are often just as upset and likely to be emotionally affected by events. It is important to recognise when it might be that the carers are also feeling the strain. This is something that all of the health professionals involved in stroke care need to try and be aware of. Sometimes carers feel guilty about admitting that they too feel unwell – as they are not the ones who have had the stroke. Anxiety is common – about whether another stroke will happen, about how to cope, finances, work, housing – the list of potential worries is a long one. Discussing and getting help from the right agencies about these problems makes it much easier to cope with them. Ultimately that benefits everyone.

Relationships
The potential impact that a stroke can have on relationships is a subject that really needs a book to itself. The occurrence of a stroke may dramatically change a couple's circumstances in every way, from their finances to their sex life. The rest of the family too are likely to have to make many adjustments. When someone who was previously healthy becomes suddenly and significantly disabled for any reason, there is a natural sense of loss that has a lot in common with a bereavement. Few if any of us plan to suddenly become a carer, or feel that it is something that we could do well at the drop of a hat.

In the early stages after someone's stroke the newness of everything that is happening, along with the uncertainty of the future, will usually produce considerable anxiety. Getting as much information as possible can help to dispel myths and show that stroke is not only a common condition but is one that most people get through successfully. Stroke support organisations and local groups can give the sort of help and support that only people who have been in the same boat can provide (see appendix C).

Many of the personal and relationship difficulties that can arise are seen repeatedly. It is good to read more about these, and discuss them with others if you can. Most people who go through a bad patch and come through it have useful tips for those who are only starting on that journey. Professional help for couples is also available. Openness about what the problems are is almost always a better policy than shutting up about them.

Specific issues such as sexual relations are often left without action for too long. Following a stroke there can be real difficulties, such as impotence in the man or a lack of libido in either or both partners. Some of those problems may in turn be related to medication, for example high blood pressure treatments quite often cause a man to have erection difficulties. A change in treatment might solve the problem; alternatively one of the modern treatments for erectile dysfunction can prove very effective. A word with the GP is all that might be needed to sort the problem out – a switched-on GP might make it easier by asking without prompting. Sex is safe after a stroke and if it was an important part of the relationship before the stroke its continuance can help to reinforce the fact that life goes on after the stroke.

7. CONTINENCE

About 50 per cent of people in the early stages after a stroke will have incontinence of urine. Incontinence of faeces is less common but even more distressing. The simple things in life are the most important, and continence is one of them. Incontinence has a marked lowering effect on a person's self-esteem and self-confidence. Its presence can contribute significantly to depression. Good incontinence treatment can matter enormously after a stroke.

When incontinence occurs it needs to be assessed and a

correctable cause found, if possible. For example, it might be an infection of the bladder and urine that responds nicely to a course of antibiotics. Similarly, incontinence of faeces might have a simple cause and solution. Bad constipation (which might be due to a combination of immobility and medication such as painkillers) can lead to loss of bowel control. The answer might involve nothing more than getting the bowel cleared out and the medication adjusted. The point is not to assume that everything is only due to the stroke.

When simple and correctable causes have been sought and treated, incontinence still remains a problem for a significant number of people. Fortunately continence support is now a well worked-out process in community care. Usually this is a matter looked after mostly by the community nurses, but each area also has an incontinence adviser (usually also a nurse) who is specially trained to advise and support the other members of the team.

Catheters

A catheter is a thin flexible tube placed in the bladder and leading out to a drainage and collecting system. Short-term use of a catheter may be needed in the early stages of a stroke if the bladder fails to drain properly or for general nursing reasons such as skin care. Catheters are best avoided in the longer term if possible but occasionally they have to be accepted. Long-term catheters have consequences, such as an increased rate of bacteria in the urine and an impact on sexual function that needs to be taken into account, particularly in younger people who have had a stroke.

8. WORK

This is another large and complex topic, and a relevant one as a quarter of all people who have a stroke are in the working age range. Whether people get back to work after a stroke depends not only on their level of disability but also on the type of job they did beforehand, their personal circumstances and many other factors that cannot be comprehensively covered here.

In the initial stages after a stroke most people will need to take a break from their job. In some occupations, such as commercial vehicle driving, there is no choice as mandatory periods are required off work, and conditions apply to whether one can return or not. The law does not cover most jobs however, and the GP is the person who normally advises on someone's fitness to return to work.

Many companies employ, directly or indirectly, an occupational health adviser. This is usually a doctor, although sometimes it may be a nurse in the first instance. They may provide advice to the employer on the employee's absence, about how long it might last and what adjustments might be required to facilitate the employee's return.

The range of benefits an employee is entitled to depends also on a person's terms of employment. Some people have protected pay for several months, others have no such protection. Most self-employed people are not covered for prolonged periods of sickness absence.

A person's entitlement to benefits is another complicated area that can take a bit of understanding. The Disability Employment Adviser in the local Jobcentre Plus office or Jobcentre will help with enquiries on employment, re-training opportunities and benefit claims. Independent advice on entitlements can be obtained from the local Citizens' Advice Bureau – these are listed in the phone directory.

Getting back to work may be a priority for some younger people who have had a stroke. Others may wish to take early retirement if it is appropriate and they can afford to. There is a good deal of useful information on work and related topics on the web sites of the main charity organisations listed in appendix C.

9. DRIVING

The Driver and Vehicle Licensing Authority (DVLA) guidance on stroke for ordinary car license holders is that you must not drive for one month after the stroke. There is no need to inform the DVLA during that period. If, however, there is any residual sign of the stroke after a month, in particular any problems with vision, higher mental functions such as concentration and understanding, or problems with limb movement, then the DVLA must be informed. The DVLA will then ask you for further information. When necessary they may need, with your permission, to contact your GP for more information.

Decisions on fitness to drive thereafter are made on an individual basis. Plenty of help and advice are available for anyone who needs to consider using an adapted vehicle following a stroke. Local authorities can provide this information, as can the main organisations listed in appendix C.

Key Points

- Combinations of disabilities are common after a stroke. For example, right-sided power loss may be accompanied by speech and language difficulties.
- Physiotherapy aims to preserve and improve lost muscle power and movement.
- Aphasia is difficulty in understanding or expressing language.
- Dysarthria is difficulty with the mechanism of speech.
- The speech and language therapist assists in diagnosing and treating problems relating to speech, language and swallowing.
- Nutrition can be impaired in stroke, mainly when there are swallowing problems, and should be attended to early on.

Treatment ranges from simple dietary modification to the use of feeding tubes.
- Change in body awareness can occur after stroke and may need special attention.
- Mood change, particularly depression, is common after stoke. It should be looked for and treated if necessary. Relationship difficulties may also arise. Counselling and support are available from the health, social and voluntary services.
- Incontinence is common after a stroke, although correctable causes should be looked for. A good deal of practical assistance is available for those with persistent incontinence after a stroke.
- A significant proportion of strokes occur in people who are in employment. The Disability Employment Adviser of the local Jobcentre should be able to provide guidance on work-related rights, disability provisions and access to benefits. Citizen's Advice Bureaux can also help.

Chapter 10

Stroke risk

Our knowledge of what causes strokes to happen is as yet incomplete. For some of the causes, such as high blood pressure, we have a reasonably good understanding of the effects this has on the body's circulation over time, and how that can lead to a stroke. There are other facts about stroke, such as that men are generally at higher risk than women, for which we can observe a link but cannot fully explain. The 'causes' of stroke are therefore really a mixture of observations that certain factors are important together with a variable level of understanding of the underlying processes going on.

On top of the specific treatments required for the individual conditions that contribute to stroke risk there are the general measures that were covered in chapter 6. In the main these are the treatments that reduce the tendency of blood to clot – the 'anti-platelet' drugs. These drugs are centrally important in reducing future stroke risk and are part of the standard treatment that everyone who has had a stroke should receive unless there are very good reasons otherwise.

Taking the broadest view of the risk factors for stroke one can divide them into two groups – those that you can do nothing about ('non-modifiable') and those that you can potentially change for the better ('modifiable').

Non-modifiable risk factors for stroke

AGE

You can't stop getting older, and old people have more strokes than young ones. For each decade in life that you get older beyond the age of 55 your stroke risk doubles. In the older age groups it is also more common to have heart disease, diabetes and other important conditions, many of which contribute significantly to stroke risk. Even when you take account of that, however, the inescapable fact is that having a stroke is one of those risks that you cannot completely avoid, so long as you live.

GENDER

Men are 25–30 per cent more likely to have a stroke than women in the age range 45 to 70. It has been thought for years that the 'protective' effect of the female hormones in women during their reproductive years is the reason for this difference but this is probably too simple an explanation – we really don't know why the difference exists. After the age of about 70 the occurrence of strokes is about equal between men and women, but because women outlive men there are more elderly women who have had a stroke than men.

ETHNIC ORIGIN

People of Afro-Caribbean and black African origin are about twice as likely to suffer a stroke than Caucasians.

HEREDITY
A small number of rare conditions exist in which the tendency to have a stroke at a younger age arises. The relationship between family history and stroke can be quite difficult to disentangle as it can be mixed up with the risk of developing other relevant conditions such as high blood pressure and diabetes, for example, which also tend to cluster in families.

PREVIOUS STROKE OR HEART ATTACK
People who have already had a stroke or a heart attack have demonstrated that they are at higher than average risk. Without treatment to reduce their risk, stroke survivors are about 15 times more likely to have another stroke compared to the 'average' population of the same age. Effective treatment of modifiable risk factors reduces the chance of another event happening.

Modifiable risk factors for stroke

Our effort must of course be concentrated on doing what we can to lower our risk of stroke. Fortunately there are many such modifiable risk factors. Most of these are the same ones that we know increase the risk of developing disease of the blood vessels of the heart (coronary heart disease). Actions taken for one are therefore doubly beneficial.

MAIN MODIFIABLE RISK FACTORS
The most important are:

- High blood pressure (hypertension)
- Smoking
- Diabetes
- High alcohol consumption
- Obesity
- Raised blood cholesterol
- Atrial fibrillation – a type of irregularity of the heartbeat

(Further details on each of these conditions are in the next chapter.)

OTHER MODIFIABLE RISK FACTORS

Other important modifiable risk factors for stroke include:

- Oral contraceptive pill. Statistically the pill is a very safe medication, used by millions of women the world over without trouble. It has also been long known to slightly increase the tendency of the blood to clot and complications such as stroke are therefore sometimes linked to its use.
- Hormone replacement therapy (HRT) uses similar types of hormones to the combined oral contraceptive pill, albeit at smaller doses, and is associated with a higher risk of stroke.
- Drug abuse. Cocaine raises the blood pressure, potentially to dangerously high levels. Weak points can exist in the arteries of the brain, in a person of any age, which are at risk of rupturing if subjected to excessively high blood pressure. Such a brain haemorrhage may prove fatal or, if not, result in a severe stroke. Intravenous drug abuse with other drugs such as heroin can also cause a stroke, either through the direct toxic effects of the drug or because of the consequences of drug abuse such as infection of the blood and damage to the heart valves. Amphetamines can also cause brain infarction and haemorrhage.

The importance of the risk factors for stroke and heart disease is increased when more than one is present. Thus a young woman on the pill who is fit, does not smoke, has a normal blood pressure, takes regular exercise, has no family history of blood clots and no other risk factors has little to be worried about. A 60-year-old man who is overweight, smokes, has high blood pressure and diabetes and takes no exercise should be very concerned.

MINORITY RISK FACTORS

Other minority risk factors for stroke exist, such as:

- Migraine. People with migraine are at about double the risk of developing stroke. This is particularly true if the pattern of the person's migraine includes visual disturbance at the start of an attack.
- Raised homocysteine levels in the blood. Homocysteine is a by-product of the body's normal metabolism but in some people with an inherited disturbance of metabolism the level of homocysteine is very high. This is associated with an increased tendency to clots in the blood. These families tend to have a history of heart attack and stroke in younger members (in their 40s and 50s). Raised levels of homocysteine in the blood of the 'normal' population are also associated with increased risk of coronary heart disease. A high intake of fruit and vegetables can possibly counteract the adverse effects of raised homocysteine.

Hardening of the arteries – 'atherosclerosis'

Although there are many potential risk factors for the development of stroke (and coronary heart disease) a common thread runs through most of them. In particular, hypertension, diabetes, smoking and raised cholesterol all increase the rate at which our arteries 'harden'. This process was referred to in chapter 2, and as it is the common pathway by which most strokes occur it is worth taking some time to explain it.

When we are young and healthy our arteries are flexible and wide, but as we get older they tend to develop thicker walls and to become less flexible. As a result, blood finds it harder to get through them. The common term for this is 'hardening of the arteries' and the proper medical term is 'atherosclerosis'.

When atherosclerosis affects the arteries of the legs then a person will have difficulty walking long distances without having to stop because of muscle aches in the calves. The aches are due to the muscles running out of nutrients such as oxygen, as the blood supply can't keep up with the muscles' needs. When the arteries of the heart get narrowed the same problem of running out of oxygen causes pain from the heart muscle, which we call angina.

Progressive narrowing of the large arteries serving the brain is a major cause of stroke. One of the main zones where atherosclerosis builds up is at junctions where arteries divide and send off branches. Chapter 7 covered the most common such occurrence as far as stroke is concerned, where furring builds up at the point where the main carotid artery in the neck divides into the internal carotid artery serving the brain and the external carotid artery serving the face (see also figures 1 and 9).

How arteries finally become blocked

THROMBOSIS

Atherosclerosis is a slow process, usually taking many years to develop, whereas a stroke occurs over minutes or hours. What seems to happen most commonly is that the surface of an area of artery affected by this 'hardening' process becomes fragile and has a tendency to break up easily. When that happens the inner lining of the artery becomes exposed, which in turn triggers the clotting action of the blood to occur over the exposed segment. This process is similar to what happens when you cut yourself. At the point of damage the body's complicated process for sealing off a cut swings into action, so a clot develops over the injury. Where the blockage occurs due to this sudden final closure of an area within an artery that's been slowly getting narrower for years we call it a thrombosis.

Figure 9: Clearing of blocked artery in the neck ('carotid endarterectomy')

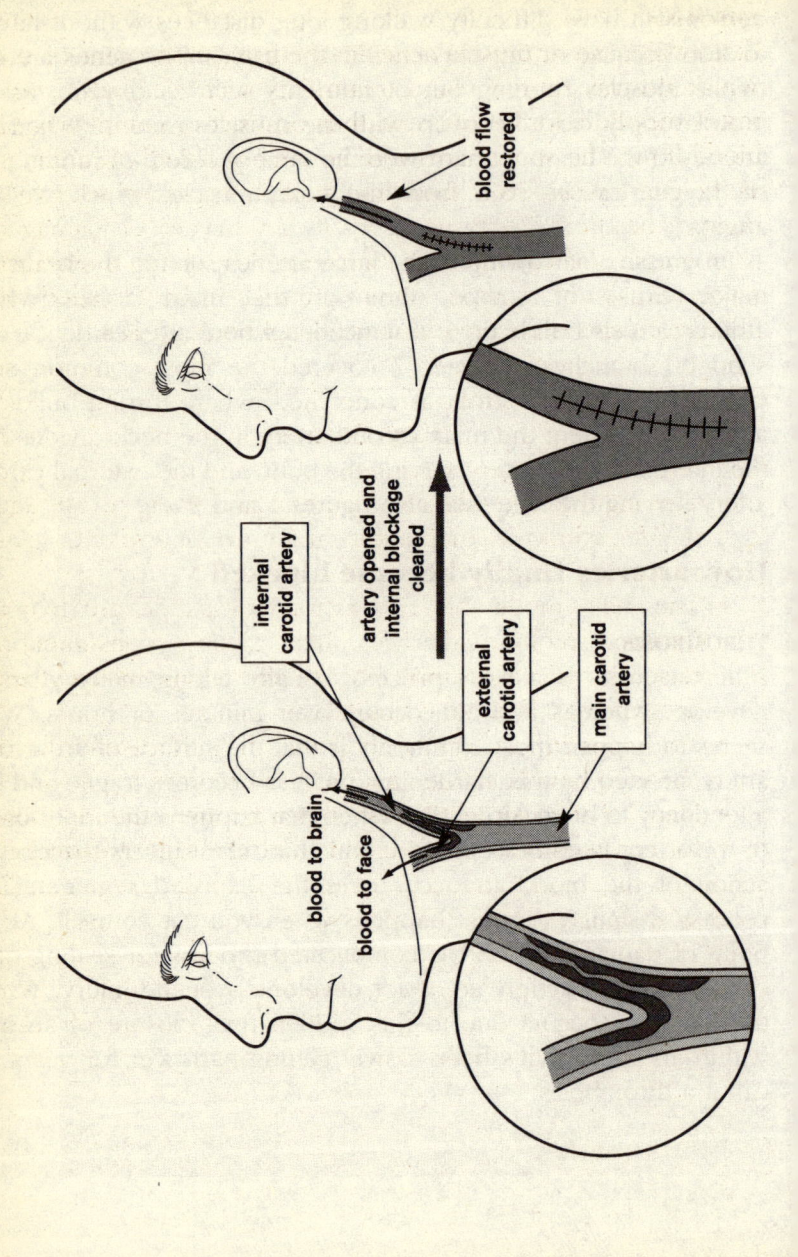

EMBOLISM

Clots within an artery may break free from their point of origin. Whisked away by the bloodstream they will eventually come to rest somewhere further on, and thus obstruct or completely block blood flow. The source could be an area of furred-up artery such as the internal carotid in the neck. Another important source is the heart, either from the heart valves if they have been damaged or from within the chambers of the heart. The latter is particularly associated with a type of irregular heartbeat called atrial fibrillation, and is covered in more detail on page 108.

Key Points

- The main non-modifiable risk factors for stroke are age, gender, ethnic origin, heredity and previous stroke or heart attack.
- The main modifiable risk factors for stroke are hypertension, smoking, diabetes, high alcohol consumption, raised blood cholesterol, obesity and a type of heartbeat irregularity called atrial fibrillation.
- The more risk factors an individual has, the likelier he or she is to have a stroke at some point in time.
- Many of the risk factors for stroke are the same as those for coronary heart disease and share the same treatments.

Chapter 11

Tackling the main modifiable risk factors for stroke

To recap, the main modifiable risk factors for stroke are high blood pressure, smoking, diabetes, high alcohol consumption, obesity, raised blood cholesterol and atrial fibrillation (a type of irregularity of the heartbeat). There is a good deal of overlap between most of these factors. People who are overweight tend to have high blood pressure and are more likely to be diabetic. High alcohol consumption pushes up the blood pressure, diabetic people need particularly good blood pressure control, and so on. Full coverage of each of these important topics is impractical in a short book of this nature but a brief summary of each follows. Other titles in the NetDoctor Help Yourself to Health series that cover the main topics in more detail are: *High Blood Pressure, How to Stop Smoking, Diabetes* and *How to Keep Healthy.*

The information presented here is relevant both to secondary prevention (i.e. action taken after someone has had their first stroke) as well as primary prevention. For those who have had a stroke the extent to which they will be able to engage with measures to reduce their risk of further stroke will depend partly on how disabled the stroke has left them. Trying to reduce the risk of stroke is always worthwhile. A little done in each of the main areas all adds up.

High blood pressure (hypertension)

WHAT IS 'BLOOD PRESSURE'?
The heart is a pump designed to force blood through the miles of piping of our blood vessels, and pumps work by generating pressure. Too much pressure puts a strain on the piping and on the pump itself, which might cause a pipe to burst or the pump to fail under the strain – in the worst case stopping altogether. Although this is a simplification, it fits with many of the observed consequences of high blood pressure.

TAKING THE BLOOD PRESSURE
To take a reading of blood pressure in the standard way the doctor or nurse wraps a cloth 'cuff' around the arm of the patient, within which is a flat rubber bladder. The bladder has two tubes coming out of it. One is connected to a small rubber bulb which, when squeezed, allows air to be pumped into the bladder. As the cloth of the cuff prevents the bladder from expanding the increased pressure goes into squeezing the person's arm. The second tube from the bladder goes to a pressure-measuring device. Historically this has been a glass column filled with mercury. Because mercury is so heavy a vertical column about 25cm tall is enough to cope with the entire range of blood pressure readings shown by human beings. By pumping up the cuff and listening to the character of the pulse as it comes through the patient's arm the doctor or nurse can read two measurements:

- The maximum pressure achieved at each heartbeat. This is called the **systolic** blood pressure.
- The minimum pressure just before the next heartbeat happens. This is called the **diastolic** blood pressure.

The traditional units of measurement for blood pressure are 'millimetres of mercury' (abbreviated to 'mmHg'). This refers to the height of the mercury column at which the systolic and diastolic readings are apparent. As mercury is a potentially toxic substance traditional blood-pressure gauges are increasingly being replaced by electronic devices that do everything automatically.

Blood pressure readings are usually written in shorthand, like this: 120/90, which means a systolic pressure of 120mmHg and a diastolic pressure of 90mmHg. Systolic and diastolic pressures can behave in different ways, which is why both readings are always taken and it is important to know both.

BLOOD PRESSURE AND THE INDIVIDUAL

Blood pressure is not constant in individuals over the course of their lives. Even those whose pressure is deemed 'normal' show a tendency for their pressure to rise with age.

This pattern of blood pressure rising with age is seen only in 'developed' countries, and probably reflects our high intake of salt, and the tendency, with age, to become overweight and inactive, with lower levels of cardiovascular fitness. At all ages until about 60 onwards men tend to have higher blood pressure than women. Elderly women, however, have slightly greater pressure than men, and are more likely to have high blood pressure too.

BLOOD PRESSURE AND POPULATIONS

Western-style diets seem to increase blood pressure with time, but there are other observed differences between population groups. Black people tend to show higher blood pressures than whites and the health problems associated with hypertension are more pronounced in the black population. Hypertension is common in Japan but results more often in stroke than in heart disease because the traditional Japanese diet is low in fat and high in salt. Japanese who move to the USA and adopt American eating habits eat more fat and less salt, and then start to show more heart disease but fewer strokes.

'HYPERTENSION'

The medical term for high blood pressure is 'hypertension'. Like most biological measurements there is no clear dividing line between high, normal and low blood pressure any more than there is an obvious distinction between tall, average or short stature. However, research has shown the levels of blood pressure above which health problems can start to arise. We know that people with systolic blood pressure consistently above 140mmHg need treatment, and those with diastolic pressure above 90mmHg do too. Both systolic and diastolic pressure are important – either one being elevated to these levels merits treatment even if the other is normal. The systolic is, however, thought to be the more important.

These are the general upper limits of blood pressure we should be trying to achieve across the population, but lower levels are desirable for most of us. The aim of blood pressure treatment is to achieve systolic pressure below 140mmHg and diastolic pressure below 85mmHg on a permanent basis. In diabetic people the thresholds are even stricter, with maximum ideal values of 130mmHg for systolic and 80mmHg for diastolic blood pressure.

If your blood pressure exceeds these ranges it does not necessarily mean that you have something to worry about. Achieving blood pressure levels low enough to be considered 'ideal' is not easy for many people and can prove impossible. The basic principle is that lower is better, and sometimes one has to compromise between the level of the blood pressure and the side effects of any treatment required to get the pressure down.

SYMPTOMS OF HIGH BLOOD PRESSURE

> The most important thing to remember about hypertension is that in the early stages it often has no symptoms. Finding out for the first time that someone has high blood pressure after they have had a stroke is finding out too late.

Unlike a joint affected by arthritis, high blood pressure causes no pain. It almost never causes headaches, despite the popular myth that it does. Someone with high blood pressure looks normal – having a 'high colour' is no guide to your blood pressure at all. You can have high blood pressure for years and feel perfectly fit and well. We all need to be aware of the need to *periodically have our blood pressure checked*, regardless of how well we feel. The majority of people with raised blood pressure are presently untreated because they don't know they've got it.

How to keep your blood pressure down

Much can be done by individuals to lower their blood pressure if it is high. This should always be the first line of treatment. Although many people who have high blood pressure need drug treatment to get their pressure down to desirable levels, they can reduce the amount of medication needed by applying the same self-help measures. Full information on the drugs used in hypertension treatment is outside the scope of this book but is detailed in the companion book in the NetDoctor series. Five ways in which blood pressure can be lowered without pills are:

1. Reduce your salt intake
2. Increase your fruit and vegetable intake
3. Avoid being overweight
4. Take regular exercise
5. Moderate your alcohol intake

SALT REDUCTION

We are a nation of salt addicts. The recommended total daily intake of salt for adults is 5 grams or less – a slightly heaped teaspoonful. Bearing in mind that this is to include all of the 'hidden' salt in processed and packaged foods, it leaves little room for the addition of salt at the table or in cooking. We can easily take two to four times as much salt as we need without trying, because so much unnecessary salt comes to us in every variety of food. Reducing salt intake to the recommended maximum can have the same effect on hypertension as powerful drug treatment. The impact is greater in adults over 45 years old and in people of African and Caribbean origin, who in general are more 'salt-sensitive'.

Leave the salt shaker off the table, and cut the amount specified in recipes by half for a start. Fast foods such as hamburgers, preserved meats and fish, sausages, bacon, soy sauce, stock cubes, pickles, crisps and similar snacks are obvious high-salt sources but bread, tinned soups, microwave meals and a host of other foods may contain more salt than you think – a single slice of bread can contain 0.5g of salt. Look for lower-salt brands. They are beginning to appear in greater numbers on supermarket shelves as the message begins to get through to the food industry that we want less salt.

FRUIT AND VEGETABLE INTAKE

Balance your vegetable intake between the orange/red and green varieties. As an easy rule the darker and brighter the colour of the vegetable the more vitamins, minerals and fibre it usually contains – compare lettuce with the deep dark green of spinach or the bright orange of carrots for example. The more starchy vegetables such as corn, butternut, pumpkin, peas, root vegetables and sweet potatoes should also be balanced with the less starchy vegetables such as courgettes, green beans, spinach, broccoli and cauliflower.

Aim for three or four portions of vegetables each day. One portion is:

- 1 cup of raw leafy vegetables
- ½ cup of other vegetables, cooked or raw
- ¾ of a cup of vegetable juice

Try eating your vegetables raw as part of a sandwich filling or serve them with dips. You can make your own dip using yoghurt and finely chopped vegetables. Try juicing vegetables – they make a refreshing drink and, once prepared, it's a quick and easy way to increase your vegetable intake.

Microwave or lightly steam vegetables when cooking, which helps retain the nutrients, and makes preparation easier and less time consuming.

To gain the maximum benefit from fruit, ensure that whenever possible it is fresh, and if the skins are edible, eat them too. Dried fruits and fruit juices can form part of your daily diet. However, they should be used in moderation, as fruit juices lose most of their natural fibre in the juicing process and dried fruits are high in carbohydrate (sugar).

Try to eat a minimum of three portions of fruit every day – more if you can. A portion of fruit is:

- 1 medium apple, orange, banana
- ½ cup chopped, cooked or canned fruit
- ¾ cup fresh fruit juice
- ¼ cup dried fruit

Combine fruits like oranges and mangos in a liquidised fruit drink. Add chopped fresh fruit to your breakfast cereal or in yoghurt as part of a mid-morning snack.

Alcohol

Consuming a small amount of alcohol daily (up to two standard units) appears to have a beneficial effect upon cardiovascular risk.

There are many possible explanations for this, but among the most likely are that compounds within some alcoholic drinks, particularly red wine, are also effective antioxidants that can neutralise 'free radical' molecules. However, the effects rapidly turn from beneficial to harmful when higher levels of alcohol are consumed. Regular alcohol consumption raises blood pressure, particularly in individuals who are already hypertensive. Binge drinking is particularly associated with an increased risk of developing a stroke.

The usual recommended maximum consumption of alcohol per week is:

- 21 units for women
- 28 units of alcohol for men

but many experts believe that more modest levels are safer:

- 14 units per week for women
- 21 units per week for men

A unit of alcohol is:

- 250ml (½ pint) of ordinary strength beer/lager
- 1 glass (125ml/4 fl oz) of wine
- 1 pub measure of sherry/vermouth (1.5oz)
- 1 pub measure of spirits (1.5oz)

Bear in mind that unmeasured home-poured spirit drinks will usually be generous, so get into the habit of using a spirit measure and sticking to it.

Obesity

Seventy per cent of the adult UK population is overweight or obese. Usually we start to put on weight after the age of 20, reaching maximum weight in middle age. Once the excess weight is put on it doesn't come off without some effort. The increase in numbers of overweight people has occurred mainly in the past two decades. During this time the total amount of food that we eat has not greatly increased, although we do now have easy access to large amounts of relatively cheap food. The main change is that we have stopped exercising.

Exercise

A lot of us kid ourselves when we estimate how much exercise we take. A couple of rounds of leisurely golf a week with liberal breaks at the nineteenth hole aren't the whole solution, although they certainly make a contribution. Similarly, people who are 'on their feet all day' but never break sweat or raise their pulse rate are helping to increase their energy expenditure but are not getting much exercise of the type that can be most useful for improving cardiovascular health.

The recommended amount of exercise that achieves health improvement is 30 minutes of brisk walking (or similar exercise) on five or six days a week. This is a slight shift away from earlier advice that promoted more vigorous, sustained activity designed to improve heart and lung function and fitness. Moderate activity, as currently recommended, also improves fitness but at a slower rate and to a lower level.

Smoking

It is impossible to keep healthy and keep smoking. Smoking just one or two cigarettes a day is proven to have health risks, as does passive smoking. All forms of tobacco smoking cause the same health problems and the only safe amount to smoke is zero. There are presently 1.1 billion people world-wide who smoke. The three most powerful factors that keep people smoking are:

1. Nicotine addiction
2. Habit formation
3. Other incentives such as peer group pressure and the effects of advertising

Of these the most important is nicotine addiction. There is quite a bit of overlap between the second and third reasons, as being in the company of a group of smokers is a prime example of a situation in which a habit will come to the surface.

QUITTING THE HABIT
More help is now available to help people quit smoking than ever before. There is a very wide range of information and support in the form of printed leaflets, on-line material, telephone help lines and internet support groups such as that on the NetDoctor web site (www.netdoctor.co.uk). Stop-smoking clinics are situated in every part of the country and you can access them either directly or through your GP. Nicotine replacement therapy (NRT) doubles the chance of someone stopping smoking and bupropion (Zyban) is another effective drug treatment suitable for some people. You can get NRT from the pharmacist but your GP can prescribe it too. Bupropion is a prescription-only medicine.

According to some stop-smoking guides it is dead easy – you just stop. Real life suggests it's a lot harder – on average people 'give up' five times before managing to quit completely.

STOPPING SMOKING ALWAYS IMPROVES HEALTH
Every time, and starting right away. No matter how much damage you think you've done to yourself, if you stop smoking you will benefit from doing so. Support information and NRT/bupropion treatment as well as advance preparation will maximise your chances of success, so it helps to get as well informed as you can before making the break. Stopping smoking is a great achievement and the last thing you want to do is to go back to square one.

However, many ex-smokers find that the desire to restart can return even years after quitting successfully. You have to consider yourself permanently vulnerable to relapse. Temptation is bound to come along... but never give in to it. One cigarette can be enough to get you started again. It's not worth it.

Diabetes

Diabetes (or diabetes mellitus to give it its full name) is the condition in which there is a raised level of glucose (sugar) in the blood. The word 'diabetes' comes from the Greek word meaning 'siphon', and refers to one of the characteristic symptoms of the condition – the passage of increased volumes of urine.

The pancreas gland, a flattish organ situated inside the abdomen, behind the stomach, controls the level of glucose circulating in the blood. It produces the hormone insulin, which is the main one that affects how glucose moves in and out of the cells of the body. Inadequate or absent production of insulin causes the type of diabetes seen usually in younger people (Type 1 diabetes), whereas in older people a different type (Type 2 diabetes) is due to resistance of the body's cells to the action of insulin. In the past few years children have been seen with Type 2 diabetes for the first time, reflecting the trend for young people to become too heavy and to be inactive. Type 2 diabetes is by far the commonest type in respect of the age group of those most affected by stroke. Treatment of Type 2 diabetes involves dietary attention (as it does also in Type 1 diabetes). When that is not enough then tablets to lower the blood glucose are required. A small proportion of people with Type 2 diabetes can also need insulin injections.

THE IMPORTANCE OF DIABETES
For reasons that we still don't fully understand, a raised blood glucose level, if present for years, can cause damage to many

tissues such as the eye, kidney and nervous system. Diabetes is the leading cause of blindness and kidney failure in the UK. Many of the problems arise because high glucose levels damage the fine structure of the arteries throughout the body. Arteries deliver the blood that nourishes every tissue and in diabetes this process is impaired. Diabetes also increases the risk of developing hardening of the arteries (atherosclerosis), which leads to narrowing and blockage of the circulation. The effects of that depend on the organ involved: blockage of heart arteries leads to angina and heart attack, whereas in the brain a stroke can result. These are much more common in diabetic people.

Fortunately, good treatment of diabetes markedly reduces the chance of serious complications developing. For treatment to be most effective, however, it is important to detect diabetes in its early stages and to treat it right away.

A significant proportion of people who are diagnosed with the commonest type of diabetes have had the condition for months or years before it is noticed. That means many already show some signs of diabetic damage before they are even started on treatment. It is therefore very important that everyone is aware of the possible signs of diabetes and that these are acted upon early.

SYMPTOMS OF DIABETES

There are several symptoms that are common to all types of diabetes:

- Thirst
- Frequent passage of urine
- Fatigue or non-specific ill health
- Blurring of vision (due to changes in the lenses of the eyes)
- Tendency to infections (particularly yeast infections like thrush)

You don't need to have all of these symptoms to be diabetic and there are many conditions other than diabetes that can cause the same symptoms. The point is that the presence of any one of them is good enough reason for you to see your doctor and have a check-up.

Raised blood cholesterol

Cholesterol is an important substance used by the body in many ways. It is a type of fat (lipid) and is the starting point of manufacture of many of the body's natural steroid hormones and of vitamin D, which is essential for the control of calcium within the body. It is also an essential component of the membrane that forms the walls of individual cells in all tissues.

Eighty per cent of the cholesterol inside us is produced by chemical processes within our own body – mostly by the liver. The amount of cholesterol we eat in our diet is of only secondary importance. Cholesterol is an important component of the fatty material that builds up in arteries in the process of atherosclerosis. This is what makes it so important in relation to strokes (and heart attacks). Lowering the amount of cholesterol in the blood has become an important part of the treatment of all diseases that arise from hardening of the arteries.

CHOLESTEROL TESTS
Cholesterol is easily measured on a blood sample and every adult should have it measured at least once before they are far past middle age. For people in whom high cholesterol runs in the family it is preferable to measure the cholesterol at a much younger age – sometime in the 20s. Cholesterol is a fairly stable measurement so if you have a normal level it does not need to be repeated for some years. If it is high then it may need quite frequent re-testing to gauge the effect of treatment.

TOTAL CHOLESTEROL
When someone quotes a single figure for their cholesterol level

they will be referring to the total cholesterol (TC). The desirable upper limit of total cholesterol (TC) is presently considered to be 4 millimoles per litre (mmol/l). As experience with the use of the main cholesterol-lowering drugs has increased over the past few years it has, however, become clear that they are of potential benefit even to people with a total cholesterol level less than 4 mmol/l.

LOWERING CHOLESTEROL

Because the bulk of the cholesterol that we have is made in the liver only a small effect can be gained by dieting. This amount is still nonetheless useful and it follows naturally when eating a healthy diet. However, a very high cholesterol level cannot be lowered sufficiently by dieting alone. A large proportion of the UK population will not achieve 'target' cholesterol levels without extra help in the form of cholesterol-lowering drug treatment. The group of drugs that have proved most useful for this purpose are called *statins*.

Statins

There are five statin drugs currently in regular use in the UK (atorvastatin, fluvastatin, pravastatin, rosuvastatin and simvastatin). All are effective at lowering cholesterol and reducing the risk of cardiovascular disease. Simvastatin happens to be the one for which the most research evidence is currently available in protecting against stroke.

> Current recommendations are that everyone who has had a stroke or TIA should take a statin if their total cholesterol level is greater than 3.5 mmol/l, unless they cannot tolerate the drug. The statin of choice is presently simvastatin, 40mg daily.

Atrial fibrillation

The heart is really made of two pumps joined together and working simultaneously. Blood returns from the body first to the right side of the heart and is then pumped through the lungs. There, fresh oxygen is taken in and carbon dioxide is released. From the lungs blood returns to the left side of the heart and is pumped out to the body again. Each half of the heart has two pumping chambers. The larger chambers, called the ventricles, do the hard work. Above each ventricle is a smaller chamber called the atrium (*plural = atria*). The atria normally contract just before the ventricles, pushing the blood they contain into the ventricles and increasing the efficiency of the heart's pumping action.

In the condition called atrial fibrillation the normal rhythmic beating of the atria is lost. Instead they beat erratically, inefficiently and out of step with the ventricles. The ventricles continue to beat in the proper way but the pulse rate is irregular, and usually rather fast. Atrial fibrillation can be a permanent finding or it can be intermittent, where periods of normal, regular beating are mingled with episodes of fibrillation. This off/on condition is called paroxysmal atrial fibrillation.

Atrial fibrillation (AF) is not a very rare condition – about 1 in 200 of the adult population have it. Underlying causes include hardening of the arteries, high blood pressure, over-activity of the thyroid gland, excessive alcohol consumption and many others. The commonest causes are more often found in older age groups, so it tends to be a condition of older people.

AF is not in itself a serious condition; in fact many people have it and are unaware of it. It does, however, have important consequences, particularly for the risk of stroke. Whereas normally blood flows through the atria and ventricles in a steady stream, the erratic beating of the atria when they fibrillate causes tiny eddy currents to form in the blood within them. In turn these can encourage the formation of small clots. The clots can then be swept into the main blood flow and travel from the left ventricle out to the rest of the body. Consequently they can get jammed in one of the smaller arteries in the brain, with familiar consequences.

On average about 5 per cent of people with atrial fibrillation have a stroke or TIA each year. At higher risk are those people who have had a previous stroke or TIA, those with high blood pressure or generally poor heart muscle function (for example following a previous heart attack), those over 65 and people with diabetes.

About one in six ischaemic strokes is associated with atrial fibrillation. This proportion rises with age to more than one in three ischaemic strokes in people over 75.

Detecting and treating AF in the many people who are presently undiagnosed is one of those many important public health targets that we still have to find ways of achieving.

TREATMENT
If an underlying cause, such as an overactive thyroid gland, is discovered and treated this may stop the AF. Usually, however, correctable causes are not found. Specialised electric shock treatment, in which the heart is briefly electrically stunned, can stop AF, but the treatment often does not work or does not last. The commonest treatment is to reduce the risk of clots forming in the blood by taking an anticoagulant drug long-term. By far the commonest drug used for this is warfarin (see appendix B). Long-term use of warfarin reduces the risk of stroke by more than two thirds.

Problems associated with warfarin include an increased risk of bleeding, which can occasionally be serious. Generally speaking the advantages of warfarin treatment in AF outweigh the disadvantages in people up to the age of 75. In people older than 75 we have less research information to guide us. We do know that the risk of serious bleeding is higher in the elderly, but even so the balance can be in favour of treatment. As with any important medical issue a decision on treatment has to be an individual matter. Not everyone with AF can take anticoagulant medicines safely, for a variety of reasons. What is important is that an informed decision is made on this matter for everyone with AF. In the majority of people warfarin treatment is appropriate and should be used.

Key Points

- The main risk factors for stroke are high blood pressure, smoking, diabetes, high alcohol consumption, obesity, raised blood cholesterol and atrial fibrillation.
- All of these risk factors interact. This means that the greater the number that are present the greater is the risk of stroke.
- It also means that a little bit of improvement in all the risk factors can add up to quite a lot of risk reduction.
- Blood cholesterol level is now less important an issue when deciding on the use of cholesterol-lowering 'statin' drugs. Almost everyone who has had a stroke or a TIA should take a statin long-term. Simvastatin is presently the recommended one but it is likely that all statins are effective at reducing stroke risk.
- Atrial fibrillation is a type of irregularity of the heartbeat. Its presence significantly increases the risk of ischaemic stroke.
- Atrial fibrillation should be treated with anticoagulant drugs (warfarin) in the majority of people.

Chapter 12

Information for carers

In general, people are not prepared for first strokes. Most strokes come unannounced. Their impact can be widespread and extend to every aspect of a person's life. The consequences of a stroke for friends, relatives and especially family can be almost as dramatic as for the patient.

There is the initial sense of shock and bewilderment about what has happened, and what is going to happen next. A stroke is a potentially life-threatening event and even if someone survives the initial days there can be much uncertainty about how much disability they will be left with. For someone still working the stroke may significantly impact on their ability to work thereafter, so financial considerations can be a source of great worry. Partners and other close contacts of the person who has had a stroke may suddenly find themselves as potential carers – a role that most feel untrained for.

Help is available

Stroke is a common medical condition and thousands of people every year must travel down the path of learning to cope with it. There is an enormous body of experience in the community, in the health and social services and in the various voluntary bodies that has been built up over decades concerning the many aspects of living after a stroke. No one wants to have a stroke in the first place but when it does happen you will find that there are many people in the same boat who can and will make it easier for you to cope. The various health professionals that come into contact with someone recovering from a stroke will do their best to ensure that all the right agencies are involved. The main voluntary organisations are particularly good sources of supportive advice in this regard (see appendix C). Through them you will also obtain contact details of local support groups. Undoubtedly there are people within a short distance of where you are who have experienced the same problems and have answers to the sort of questions you'd most like to ask. They too will know about the services that are available in your area and how best to access them.

Remember also that help can be brought to you in your own home if that's necessary, or if it is what you would prefer, both from the 'official' services and from the voluntary sector. Everyone is entitled to a full assessment of their needs, and that includes the carers' needs. That assessment is very important in shaping the type and amount of help that you are entitled to.

Information helps

Not knowing what's going on is one of the most unsettling aspects of a totally new situation. Getting a grip on the facts takes away much of the helplessness you might feel at the start. Books like this hopefully serve some purpose in trying to explain the nature of stroke, and in particular what can be done to reduce the risk of another one occurring. There is a wealth of information now available on stroke from local health services and voluntary organisations that explains in more detail many of the common issues. Full lists of their publications are obtainable from these organisations and their telephone helpline may help fill in any missing details. Ultimately, of course, what you need are the answers to the questions particular to you. Never be reluctant to ask questions of your GP, consultant, nurse, social worker, voluntary worker or anyone else involved in trying to help you. All of these people recognise the value of good quality information and want to make sure that you have what you need in that regard.

Psychological and emotional effects of stroke

Caring for a loved one who has had a stroke can be an emotional roller coaster. At times it is sad, at other times it can be funny. It is usually hard work and can often cause many conflicting feelings, including guilt, anger and frustration, but hopefully also a sense of achievement and pride at times. Relationships are often imperfect even when both partners are in good health, and one partner becoming unwell doesn't mean that everything sorts itself out.

Strokes can affect someone's emotional state. Sometimes this causes the person who has had the stroke to show changes in mood that are more intense than previously, or at times seem inappropriate. Thus he or she might burst out laughing or crying without any apparent reason. Swearing might happen without apparent restraint or in the 'wrong' circumstances. This happens if the stroke somehow disconnects someone's real mood and their means of showing it. Once everyone understands that emotional outbursts may be part of the individual pattern produced by someone's stroke then they become easier to deal with.

This does not mean of course that real mood swings do not

occur. They certainly do, and not only in the person who has had the stroke. Carers can also become depressed and anxious just as easily. The burden of caring can be a heavy one and one of the most positive things you can do as a carer is to say when you feel that you too need some extra care and attention. Bottling up your feelings leads to more stress and eventually more problems. Any of the health professionals with whom you come into contact will be alert to such problems and can discuss your feelings with you in confidence.

Reactions to long-term illness

When someone develops such an important condition as a stroke the reactions a carer goes through are similar in many ways to those of bereavement. First feelings may be more of anger than anything else – why me? Why us? You may become frustrated at the uncertainty of the outlook. Despite the improvements that are occurring in stroke care there are gaps in the availability of services across the UK, and these may be very frustrating for you. The realities of stroke treatment may seem to offer little in the way of improvements, and there are certainly no cures.

Some of that anger might be directed at the health professions but some of it may also be aimed at the person who has had the stroke. You might assume prematurely that your life with your partner is effectively over or you might worry that he or she will deteriorate further. The overwhelming nature of your early thoughts about stroke are therefore likely to be negative.

Guilt may come because you worry that you are not doing enough to help your partner or because you didn't sort out relationship problems in the past. The same feeling might come later if a move to residential care becomes necessary. The latter may come very close to the experience of losing the person as if they had died.

Getting as much of the right information and help early is the key to surviving these potentially rocky times.

Look after yourself

Your own health, both mental and physical, is going to be all the more important as your role as carer becomes more prominent over the years, so it is wise to ask your doctor for a check-up. We've mentioned that depression and anxiety are more common in carers of people with long-term illness than in the average population. Having a dependent partner does not make you immune from having your own health needs. If your GP is not the same doctor who is caring for the person who had the stroke make sure that you tell them what your home circumstances are. GPs know the system in their area, what sorts of services are available and who the right people are to get things organised.

Take breaks

One of the most important parts of caring is not caring – i.e. you need to get a break from it regularly. This could be when a volunteer comes into the house for a couple of hours once a week to let you get to the shops or have a coffee with a friend, or it might mean that your partner goes into respite care for a few weeks every now and then to let you have a bigger break. Every part of the country has some facilities available to give carers respite breaks and you are entitled to have access to those facilities.

If a stroke has left your partner significantly disabled then holidays together certainly need more planning. Travel arrangements for disabled people are improving but can be very patchy abroad. Holiday insurance requirements may apply – always ensure that you declare any disabilities in advance of travel and obtain adequate insurance cover for emergencies. There are many well-organised and resourced organisations and venues in the UK that cope well for people with different degrees of disability. The main charity organisations are useful sources of this information.

If there is a perfect carer out there somewhere who never loses their temper with their partner who has had a stroke, who never harbours any feelings of resentment, anger or self-pity about what they have to cope with, and who never feels guilty about wishing it had all turned out otherwise, then good luck to them, but they must be very few and far between. Most of us have to live with the fact that we are not perfect, and there is no shame in that.

Keep positive

Strokes can and do change lives. This does not mean that life has to come to a halt. A stroke can force a rethink of what life is about, and what one really needs to enjoy it. Small targets and successes can become more important than the grand designs of the pre-stroke era. That strokes occur is a fact of life. We may be able to reduce our risk of stroke, but we will never be able to stop strokes happening at all. There is nothing to be gained by looking back on the times before a stroke and wishing you had lived some aspects of your life differently.

Accepting what cannot be changed is one of those tasks in life that is easy to say but hard to do. Fine words are of little help when the going is tough. It's true, though, that having a positive outlook and working at emphasising the good in any situation does pay off. You can never change the past, but you can make a difference to the future.

Key Points

- Stroke, like any serious long-term medical condition, can have a major impact on family, friends and relationships.
- Few of us are well prepared for such an event. For almost everyone there is a steep hill of new learning and adaptation to climb.
- There is a great deal of advice, information and practical help available to anyone directly or indirectly affected by stroke through health, social and voluntary channels.
- It helps to learn as much as you can about stroke. Ask all the questions that it will help you to be answered.
- Caring is a hard job at the best of times. You will need and should make use of regular breaks of one sort or another.

Appendix A

References

National guidelines

- National Clinical Guidelines for Stroke (Royal College of Physicians of London); http://www.rcplondon.ac.uk/pubs/books/stroke/stroke_guidelines_2ed.pdf
- Management of Patients with Stroke (Guideline 64, Scottish Intercollegiate Guidelines Network); http://www.sign.ac.uk/guidelines/fulltext/64/index.html
- Care After Stroke Patient and Carer booklet; http://www.rcplondon.ac.uk/pubs/books/stroke/stroke_patientcarer_2ed.pdf
- National Audit Office. Reducing Brain Damage: Faster Access to Better Stroke Care; www.nao.org.uk/publications/nao_reports/05–06/0506452es.pdf

Stroke Management

- http://www.clinicalevidence.com/ceweb/conditions/cvd/0201/0201.jsp
- http://www.besttreatments.co.uk/btuk/conditions/5966.html

Stroke Prevention

http://www.clinicalevidence.com/ceweb/conditions/cvd/0207/0207.jsp
http://www.besttreatments.co.uk/btuk/conditions/10381.html

Atrial fibrillation

- Hart, R. G. and Benavente, O., Primary prevention of stroke in patients with atrial fibrillation (Royal College of Physicians of Edinburgh Consensus Conference on Atrial Fibrillation in Hospital and General Practice, July 1999); http://www.rcpe.ac.uk/publications/articles/Supplement6_%20Atrial_fibrillation/PrimaryPrevention.pdf

Carotid endarterectomy

- http://omni.ac.uk/browse/mesh/D016894.html
- http://www.sign.ac.uk/pdf/sign14.pdf

Appendix B

Drugs used in the treatment or prevention of stroke

The following information contains selected details of some of the medications used in treating or preventing stroke. Full details are included in the manufacturer's data sheets and can also be viewed within the medicines section of the NetDoctor web site: http://www.netdoctor.co.uk/medicines/

The information is accurate at the time of writing but new information on medicines appears regularly. A health professional should always be consulted concerning the prescription and use of medicines.

Medicines and their possible side effects can affect individual people in different ways. The following lists some of the side effects that are known to be associated with these medicines. Side effects other than those listed may exist.

Aspirin

Acetylsalicylic acid, otherwise known as aspirin, belongs to a group of medicines called non-steroidal anti-inflammatory drugs (NSAIDs). It works by blocking the action of an enzyme called cyclo-oxygenase. Cyclo-oxygenase is involved in the production of various chemicals in the body. These are known as prostaglandins, prostacyclins and thromboxane.

Aspirin prevents the blood cells called platelets from producing thromboxane. Thromboxane is one of the chemicals that cause platelets to clump together and start off the process of blood clotting. Stopping its production reduces the likelihood of clots forming in the blood.

High doses of aspirin (300mg and over) also prevent the production of prostaglandins. Prostaglandins are produced in response to injury or certain diseases and would otherwise go on to cause pain, swelling and inflammation. Higher doses of aspirin are therefore used to relieve pain and inflammation.

MAIN SIDE EFFECTS
- Indigestion or abdominal discomfort
- Allergic reactions such as skin rash, swelling of the lips, tongue and throat (angioedema) or narrowing of the airways (bronchospasm)
- Ulceration or bleeding of the stomach or intestines

INTERACTIONS WITH OTHER MEDICINES
Aspirin may clash with a number of other types of medicine. People taking anticoagulant medicines used to prevent blood clotting, e.g. warfarin, should not also take aspirin. This is because the higher doses of aspirin used for pain relief can irritate the stomach lining, as well as increasing the effects of warfarin, both of which increase the likelihood of bleeding. Lower doses of aspirin used for a blood-thinning effect are safer, but should

only be used by people taking anticoagulants on the advice of a doctor.

There is an increased risk of side effects if aspirin is taken with other non-steroidal anti-inflammatory drugs (NSAIDs), e.g. ibuprofen, diclofenac, indometacin. For this reason, aspirin should not be taken with any other NSAID. Low-dose aspirin used for anti-blood-clotting purposes is an exception to this, but should only be used with other NSAIDs on the instruction of a doctor.

Clopidogrel

Clopidogrel (hydrogen sulphate) is a type of medicine called an antiplatelet (sometimes referred to as a blood-thinning medicine). It stops the blood cells called platelets from clumping together and forming blood clots.

MAIN SIDE EFFECTS
- Headache
- Rash
- Itching
- Disturbances of the gut such as diarrhoea, constipation, nausea, vomiting or abdominal pain
- Bruising and bleeding
- Dizziness or balance problems involving the inner ear (vertigo)
- Pins and needles sensation
- Decrease in the number of a type of white blood cell (neutrophil) in the blood
- Decrease in the number of platelets in the blood
- Ulceration or bleeding of the stomach or intestines

INTERACTIONS WITH OTHER MEDICINES
There may be an increased risk of bleeding if clopidogrel is taken with the following medicines, which also affect blood clotting:

- aspirin
- non-steroidal anti-inflammatory drugs (NSAIDs), e.g. naproxen, ibuprofen, diclofenac
- heparin
- warfarin (not recommended for use in combination with clopidogrel).

Brand name: Plavix®

Dipyridamole slow release

Dipyridamole is another type of antiplatelet agent. It works by inhibiting the action of an enzyme found in platelets called phosphodiesterase.

Inside the platelets phosphodiesterase normally breaks down a chemical called cyclic AMP. Cyclic AMP plays a key role in blood clotting. If the level of cyclic AMP in the platelets is high this prevents the platelets from clumping together. Dipyridamole causes the levels of cyclic AMP in the platelets to rise, because it stops phosphodiesterase from breaking it down. This means that dipyridamole stops the platelets from clumping together and causing a blood clot.

MAIN SIDE EFFECTS
- Throbbing headache (normally disappears with long-term use)
- Faster than normal heart beat
- Low blood pressure
- Indigestion
- Dizziness
- Nausea and vomiting
- Hot flushes
- Pain in the muscles
- Temporary worsening of chest pain (angina) at the start of therapy
- Diarrhoea

INTERACTIONS WITH OTHER MEDICINES
Dipyridamole enhances the anti-clotting effect of the following medicines:

- other antiplatelet medicines, e.g. low-dose aspirin, clopidogrel
- anticoagulants, e.g. warfarin.

The absorption of dipyridamole from the gut may be reduced if it is taken at the same time as antacids.

Brand name: Persantin Retard®

Alteplase

Alteplase belongs to a group of medicines known as fibrinolytics. It works by attaching to a blood clot and stimulating extra production of a substance produced naturally by the body called plasmin. Plasmin is produced in the blood to break down the major constituent of blood clots (fibrin), thereby dissolving clots once they have fulfilled their purpose in stopping bleeding.

Alteplase needs to be given by injection.

MAIN SIDE EFFECTS
- Heart beat rhythm disturbances
- Low blood pressure
- Increased tendency to bleed
- Fever
- Nausea and vomiting
- An extreme allergic reaction (anaphylaxis)

Brand name: Alteplase®

Warfarin

Warfarin (sodium) is a type of medicine called an anticoagulant. Blood clots normally only form to stop bleeding that has occurred as a result of injury to the tissues. The clotting process is complicated and begins when blood cells called platelets clump together at the site of damage and produce chemicals that activate clotting factors in the blood.

Clotting factors are proteins that are produced by the liver. Vitamin K is essential for their production. The activated clotting factors cause a protein called fibrin to be converted into another called fibrinogen. Fibrinogen binds the platelets together, forming a blood clot. Warfarin works by preventing the vitamin K dependent production of the clotting factors described above. Warfarin prevents the production of these clotting factors by inhibiting the action of vitamin K. Without these clotting factors fibrin cannot be converted into fibrinogen and blood clots are therefore less likely to occur.

Warfarin takes about three days to produce its full anticoagulant effect because, while it prevents the production of new clotting factors, it takes about this long for clotting factors that have already been produced to be used up.

The anticoagulant effect of warfarin is measured by a blood test, the result of which is a number known as the INR (International Normalised Ratio). An INR in the range 2–3.5 is aimed for in the majority of people who take warfarin. Regular blood samples to measure the INR are necessary when taking warfarin. From the INR result the doctor can then judge the correct dose of warfarin to take until the next INR check.

USE WITH CAUTION

Extra care when participating in physical activities is necessary while taking warfarin, as even minor injury may result in bleeding/bruising.

As warfarin works by inhibiting the action of vitamin K, changes to your dietary intake of vitamin K can alter the effect of your warfarin. For this reason, avoid making sudden major changes to your diet, particularly your consumption of green tea, salad and green vegetables (e.g. broccoli, Brussels sprouts, or spinach), which contain large amounts of vitamin K. Large amounts of green vegetables (more than 500g daily) can reduce the effect of warfarin and should be avoided. Changes to your consumption of fats and oils can also alter the effect of warfarin, as vitamin K is a fat-soluble vitamin. Some vitamin supplements contain vitamin K and can reduce the effect of warfarin.

Other foods that can influence warfarin's effect include soya bean products, avocados and large amounts of ice cream (over a litre a day). Cranberry juice should be avoided, as should large amounts of alcohol, as these may increase the effect of warfarin. Warfarin's effect can also be altered by sudden increases or decreases in your body weight.

Consult your doctor immediately if you experience any bruising, bleeding, dark stools, blood in the urine, vomiting, diarrhoea, fever or acute illness while taking this medicine, so that your INR can be checked.

MAIN SIDE EFFECTS
Common:
- Bruising and an increased tendency to bleed

Rare:
- Diarrhoea
- Nausea and vomiting
- Rash
- Jaundice
- Hair loss

INTERACTIONS WITH OTHER MEDICINES

The anticoagulant effect of warfarin can be affected by many medicines. Always check with a pharmacist or doctor before taking any non-prescription medicines with warfarin.

The following is a selection of drugs that may enhance the effect of warfarin (increased INR; warfarin dose may need reducing):

- allopurinol
- amiodarone
- antibiotic medicines (e.g. amoxicillin, ampicillin, ciprofloxacin, erythromycin, metronidazole)
- aspirin
- cimetidine
- dipyridamole
- non-steroidal anti-inflammatory drugs (NSAIDs, particularly azapropazone, diclofenac, flurbiprofen, indometacin, phenylbutazone, piroxicam. NSAIDs may also irritate the stomach and intestinal lining, which can result in bleeding from the gut in people taking warfarin).
- omeprazole
- tamoxifen
- thyroxine (levothyroxine)

The following is a selection of medicines that may reduce the effect of warfarin (decreased INR; warfarin dose may need increasing):

- azathioprine
- carbamazepine
- oestrogens
- progestogens
- raloxifene
- St John's wort (*Hypericum perforatum*, herbal remedy)
- vitamin K

Simvastatin

Simvastatin is one of a group of drugs commonly known as 'statins'. They block the action of the enzyme HMG-CoA reductase, which is involved in the biochemical process within the body that manufactures cholesterol. Statins therefore lower the concentration of cholesterol in the blood. They also reduce the concentration of another type of fat, triglyceride, in the blood.

Statins have an important role in the prevention of strokes and heart disease as they reduce the risk of cholesterol being deposited in the major blood vessels of the heart (as well as in other parts of the body).

MAIN SIDE EFFECTS
- Headache
- Rash
- Disturbances of the gut such as flatulence, diarrhoea, constipation, nausea, vomiting or abdominal pain
- Inflammation of the pancreas
- Hair loss
- Alteration in blood tests of liver function and inflammation of the liver
- Pins and needles in the limbs
- Dizziness
- Low red blood cell count (anaemia)
- Muscle pain, weakness and breakdown

INTERACTIONS WITH OTHER MEDICINES
There may be an increased risk of muscle damage if simvastatin is taken with any of the following medicines:

- ciclosporin
- fibrates (e.g. gemfibrozil)
- nicotinic acid

- itraconazole
- ketoconazole
- erythromycin
- clarithromycin
- HIV protease inhibitors (e.g. nelfinavir)
- nefazadone

The 'blood thinning' or anti-clotting effect of anticoagulants such as warfarin may be increased when taken with simvastatin. This should be monitored when first starting treatment with simvastatin and when doses are altered.

Brand name: Zocor®

Appendix C

Useful contacts

The Stroke Association

The Stroke Association is the main stroke-related charity in England and Wales. It funds research into prevention, treatment and better methods of rehabilitation, and helps stroke patients and their families directly through its community services. These include dysphasia support, family support, information services and welfare grants. It also works to increase knowledge of stroke at all levels of society and to act as a voice for everyone affected by stroke.

The Stroke Association produces a large number of publications including patient leaflets, Stroke News (a quarterly magazine) and information for health professionals. Information leaflets are available in several languages. There is an extensive database of links on the Stroke Association web site to other useful services.

Telephone: Stroke helpline 0845 3033 100 (open Monday to Friday, 9am to 5pm)

E-mail: info@stroke.org.uk
Web: http://www.stroke.org.uk
Address: Stroke Information Service
The Stroke Association
240 City Road
London EC1V 2PR

Chest, Heart and Stroke Scotland

Chest, Heart and Stroke Scotland provides care and support throughout Scotland. Their main community service, the Volunteer Stroke Service (VSS), offers rehabilitation and support to people affected by stroke, particularly those with communication problems. The CHSS Advice Line offers confidential, professional advice from trained nurses on all aspects of chest, heart and stroke illness. Additionally there are booklets, factsheets and videos available free to patients and carers.

Telephone: 0131 225 6963
Advice helpline: 0845 077 6000
E-mail: admin@chss.org.uk
Web: http://www.chss.org.uk
Address: (Head Office)
65 North Castle Street
Edinburgh EH2 3LT

Northern Ireland Chest Heart and Stroke Association

Telephone: 028 9032 0184
Advice Helpline: 0845 769 7299
Web: http://www.nichsa.com
Address: 22 Great Victoria Street
Belfast BT2 7LX

Different Strokes

Different Strokes is a registered charity providing a unique, free service to younger stroke survivors throughout the United Kingdom. It is run by stroke survivors for stroke survivors. The web site has links to information on a number of topics, including:

- Information On Services For Stroke Survivors (services & organisations that may be able to help)
- Benefits (entitlements)
- The Invisible Side of Stroke (dealing with counselling & the emotional aspect of stroke)
- Charities That May Be Able To Assist Financially
- How To Get Help From Social Services (entitlements & procedures)
- Sex After A Stroke
- Work After Stroke

Telephone: 0845 130 7172
E-mail: info@differentstrokes.co.uk
Web: http://www.differentstrokes.co.uk
Address: Different Strokes
9 Canon Harnett Court
Wolverton Mill
Milton Keyes MK12 5NF

The Disabled Living Foundation

The Disabled Living Foundation (DLF) provides free and impartial advice and information on over 15,000 pieces of equipment, large and small, from bath seats and wheelchairs to jar openers and tap turners. Their Equipment Demonstration Centre has one of the largest displays of equipment in the UK.

Telephone: 0845 130 9177
Text phone: 020 7432 8009
E-mail: advice@dlf.org.uk
Web: http://www.dlf.org.uk

Motoring and transport

The Directgov web site provides easy access to a wide range of government information and services. Within the motoring and transport section is a large number of helpful relevant links.

Main site: http://www.direct.gov.uk/Homepage/fs/en
Motor and transport: http://tinyurl.com/9j8nq

The Continence Foundation

The Continence Foundation is a charity set up to provide information, advice and expertise about bladder and bowel problems.

Telephone: Helpline: 0845 345 0165 (Monday to Friday, 9:30am to 1pm)
Office: 020 7404 6875
E-mail: continence-help@dial.pipex.com
Address: The Continence Foundation
307 Hatton Square
16 Baldwins Gardens
London ECIN 7RJ